COMPLEMENTARY AND ALTERNATIVE MEDICINE

Complementary and Alternative Medicine is a sociological investigation of complementary and alternative medicine (CAM) in contemporary society, and an exploration of the forces throughout the globe, across different institutions, and within different therapeutic spaces, that constrain or foster alternative medicine.

Drawing on 30 years of research, the book identifies the trends in the use of CAM and explores the scientific, political and social challenges that CAM faces in relation to orthodox medicine. The author examines the varieties of CAM practices and how they manifest in different institutional spaces – including public inquiries, the orthodox medical practitioner's consulting room, medical journals and the homes of those who use CAM. It also compares unorthodox practices in different geo-political settings, namely the global north and the global south.

This book is valuable reading for higher-level undergraduate and postgraduate social science students, including those in psychology, sociology, anthropology, health sciences and related disciplines. It is relevant for courses in medical sociology, medical anthropology and social science and health, and a broader audience interested in contemporary health issues, controversies and alternative medicine.

Kevin Dew is Professor of Sociology at Victoria University of Wellington. He is a founding member of the Applied Research on Communication in Health (ARCH) group. His books include *The Cult and Science of Public Health: A Sociological Investigation* and *Public Health, Personal Health and Pills: Drug Entanglements and Pharmaceuticalised Governance*. His current research activities include studies of cancer survivorship and cancer care decision-making in relation to health inequities.

Critical Approaches to Health

Series Editors: Kerry Chamberlain & Antonia Lyons

The Routledge *Critical Approaches to Health* series aims to present critical, interdisciplinary books around psychological, social and cultural issues related to health. Each volume in the series provides a critical approach to a particular issue or important topic, and is of interest and relevance to students and practitioners across the social sciences. The series is produced in association with the International Society of Critical Health Psychology (ISCHP).

Titles in the series

Disability and Sexual Health
A Critical Exploration of Key Issues
Poul Rohleder, Stine Hellum Braathen and Mark T. Carew

Postfeminism and Health
Critical Psychology and Media Perspectives
Sarah Riley, Adrienne Evans, and Martine Robson

Health at Work
Critical Perspectives
Leah Tomkins and Katrina Pritchard

Complementary and Alternative Medicine
Containing and Expanding Therapeutic Possibilities
Kevin Dew

For more information about this series, please visit: www.routledge.com/Critical-Approaches-to-Health/book-series/CRITHEA

COMPLEMENTARY AND ALTERNATIVE MEDICINE

Containing and Expanding Therapeutic Possibilities

Kevin Dew

Routledge
Taylor & Francis Group
LONDON AND NEW YORK

ISCHP
International Society of
Critical Health Psychology

First published 2021
by Routledge
2 Park Square, Milton Park, Abingdon, Oxon OX14 4RN

and by Routledge
605 Third Avenue, New York, NY 10158

Routledge is an imprint of the Taylor & Francis Group, an informa business

British Library Cataloguing-in-Publication Data
A catalogue record for this book is available from the British Library

Library of Congress Cataloging-in-Publication Data
A catalog record for this book has been requested

ISBN: 978-0-367-25321-9 (hbk)
ISBN: 978-0-367-25323-3 (pbk)
ISBN: 978-0-429-28717-6 (ebk)

Typeset in Bembo
by Apex CoVantage, LLC

ACKNOWLEDGEMENTS

My thanks to Kerry Chamberlain and Antonia Lyons for giving me the opportunity to build on my interests in sociology of CAM by inviting me to write for this book series. I am indebted to many great research colleagues, far too many to mention, who have supported me over the years, and to the many research participants who have contributed so much to my understanding of health practices. I would like to thank Rick Weiss for his suggestions for Chapter 6, and I am grateful to the School of Social and Cultural Studies at Victoria University of Wellington for providing me with the institutional home that has been so accommodating to my academic endeavours.

CONTENTS

Series editor preface *viii*
Antonia Lyons & Kerry Chamberlain

1 Introduction to complementary and alternative medicine and therapeutic pluralism 1

2 State medicine, regulating practices and the creation of alternatives 10

3 Disciplining and integrating practices 26

4 Adjusting to statist medicine and the manipulation of chiropractic 46

5 Transformation, continuity and the ebb and flow of Chinese medicine 63

6 Empire, tradition and the many therapeutic faces of India 84

7 The CAM user and the expansion of therapeutic possibilities 102

8 The fraught use of CAM in cancer care 121

9 Incoherent forces: the disciplining and the unruliness of complementary and alternative therapies 140

Index *149*

SERIES EDITOR PREFACE

Critical Approaches to Health

Health is a major issue for people all around the world and is fundamental to individual well-being, personal achievements and satisfaction, as well as to families, communities and societies. It is also embedded in social notions of participation and citizenship. Much has been written about health, from a variety of perspectives and disciplines, but a lot of this writing takes a biomedical and causally positivist approach to health matters, neglecting the historical, social and cultural contexts and environments within which health is experienced, understood and practiced. It is timely for a new series of books that offer critical, social science perspectives on important health topics.

The *Critical Approaches to Health* series aims to provide new critical writing on health by presenting critical, interdisciplinary and theoretical writing about health, where matters of health are framed quite broadly. The series seeks to include books that range across important health matters, including general health-related issues (such as gender and media), major social issues for health (such as medicalisation, obesity and palliative care), particular health concerns (such as pain, doctor-patient interaction, health services and health technologies), particular health problems (such as diabetes, autoimmune disease and medically unexplained illness) or health for specific groups of people (such as the health of migrants, the homeless and the aged) or combinations of these.

The series seeks above all to promote critical thought about health matters. By critical, we mean going beyond the critique of the topic and work in the field, to more general considerations of power and benefit, and in particular, to addressing concerns about whose understandings and interests are upheld and whose are marginalised by the approaches, findings and practices in these various domains of health. Such critical agendas involve reflections on what constitutes knowledge, how it is created and how it is used. Accordingly, critical approaches consider epistemological and theoretical positioning, as well as issues of methodology and practice, and seek to examine how health is enmeshed within broader social relations and structures. Books within this series take up this challenge and seek to provide new insights and understandings by applying a critical agenda to their topics.

In this book, *Complementary and Alternative Medicine: Containing and Expanding Therapeutic Possibilities*, Kevin Dew interrogates the place of complementary and alternative medicine (CAM) in contemporary society. He provides valuable overviews of the terminology and understandings of the concept of CAM, documenting how CAM has increased in popularity over the last few decades and has an important place in healthcare around the world. In shining a light on complementary approaches (those that sit alongside and help conventional medicine) and alternative approaches (those that might be in opposition to conventional medicine), we learn a lot about dominant/conventional medicine and therapeutic healing systems. As the author points out early in this book, 'there may be little that unifies CAM', although throughout the remainder of the book he shows that there are similarities in some of the more historical and organised CAM approaches in terms of their understandings of the nature of disease, bodies and health.

Throughout the book, there is an emphasis on providing critical insights into the relationship between CAM and orthodox medicine in many different geolocative, social, cultural and political contexts. Research and evidence is drawn on to identify and argue for how CAM practice, uptake and understandings are shaped by social, political and historical forces in different nation-states. This broad, critical overview allows the author to convincingly convey the diversity, complexity and ongoing change around CAM. Alongside this, specific case studies are employed to demonstrate how biomedicine has shaped and disciplined those healing practices that become credible and legitimate. This includes the histories and practices of specific CAM approaches (and the experiences of practitioners and clients), including chiropractic and traditional Chinese medicine (TCM).

This book offers a thoughtful, accessible, engaging and up-to-date account of the tensions – and opportunities – that surround CAM in different places around the world. The book clearly articulates, through grounded examples, how therapeutic practices are shaped by dominant societal and political forces and how nothing remains static in these spaces of treatment and healing. The book articulates the key tensions that play out in relation to therapeutic practices that are supported by the state and its institutions, and those that are marginalised, and what this ultimately means for people, practitioners and our understandings of healing. Thus, the book offers the reader a thought-provoking – and at times unsettling – consideration of the power and structure of contemporary healing systems. As such, it makes an excellent and original addition to the *Critical Approaches to Health* series.

Antonia Lyons & Kerry Chamberlain
October 2020

1

INTRODUCTION TO COMPLEMENTARY AND ALTERNATIVE MEDICINE AND THERAPEUTIC PLURALISM

This book focuses on therapeutic approaches that are not dominant. A clumsy phrasing might then be non-dominant therapeutic systems. What currently dominates globally is often given a shorthand of 'biomedicine', which gives something of the flavour of a biologically based system of therapeutics, and so disease and illness are reduced to biological causes. Treatment is meant to correct an injury of a specific process that is causing the illness – so insulin for diabetes, antibiotics for an infection, bypass surgery for the heart and so on. The body may be treated as if it functions like a machine. Objective, rational, detached care is what is required.

Non-dominant systems then do things other than this. They may be biologically based but there will be other components that are not part of dominant therapeutic thinking. Rather than a machine metaphor being used the body might be considered as a vital organism in which different bodily forces are in dynamic equilibrium. Instead of a specific treatment to deal with some specific symptoms or signs, treatment might be addressed to the whole person. Instead of being rational and detached, some approaches might acknowledge intuition and rapport.

A common term used to describe this collection of non-dominant therapeutic systems is complementary and alternative medicine (CAM). CAM has an important place in healthcare throughout the world, and in many countries, its popularity has been on the increase over the last few decades. The interest in CAM extends to international organisations, with the World Health Organization outlining a Traditional Medicine Strategy 2014–2023 to facilitate the development of regulations on CAM and integration of CAM into national health systems (Pokladnikova and Telec 2020). The term complementary suggests approaches that help with the healing of dominant medicine. The term alternative suggests a different way of doing things that could potentially be in opposition to dominant medicine. Other terms include heterodox systems that are then opposed to an orthodox system. Unconventional medicine perhaps, but unconventional to what (Jütte 2001)? In France, the term médicines parallèles is used, so suggesting different therapeutic systems that do not actually meet, but are in parallel (Herzlich 2001).

Researchers of CAM use a great variety of definitions, and some are rather loose and vague, such as therapies that patients use along with conventional therapies (Roberts et al. 2006), and healthcare practices that are not part of their country's own traditional or conventional medicine (Pokladnikova and Telec 2020).

The National Center for Complementary and Alternative Medicine (2000) in the United States classifies CAM into the following domains:

1 Alternative medical systems, such as traditional Chinese medicine (TCM), ayurveda and homeopathy, that developed independently from biomedicine.
2 Mind-body interventions, which aim to support the mind to enhance bodily function, including meditation and dance therapy.
3 Biologically based therapies and dietary approaches, including herbalism and vitamin supplementation.
4 Manipulation and body-based therapies, which work on the physical body of the patient and include chiropractic, osteopathy and massage.
5 Energy therapies, which work on energy fields in or around the body and include reiki and therapeutic touch.

Scholars categorise CAM and unconventional medicine in different ways. For example, Robert Jütte suggests four categories: physical therapies such as chiropractic, biological therapies such as homeopathy, nutritional therapies and spiritual therapies such as healing touch (Jütte 2001). As such, there may be little that unifies CAM.

However, even given this diversity some of the more organised and historically rooted CAM approaches can have similar understandings of the nature of disease, bodies and health. Systems as diverse as homeopathy originating in Germany, Japanese Kampō, siddha in India and many others do not necessarily approach treatment decision making in terms of diagnosing a disease. Rather, they attempt to find the right treatment for the individual, and so the disease name does not lead to the preferred remedy in a straightforward manner. Kampō doctors regard each patient as having a unique illness for which a unique treatment is required, which may include a specific mixture of herbs with acupuncture. The diagnosis is not a process of labelling the illness but is focused on cure – what needs to be given for this person (Ohnuki-Tierney 1997). Similar understandings underlie homeopathy and siddha, as will be discussed in later chapters. Whereas Western medicine may focus on the malfunctioning of a physiological process with the treatment directed at that process, some CAM approaches focus on the suffering person (Cunningham and Andrews 1997). Despite rhetorical gestures towards patient-centred medicine and patient empowerment, the patient's input into the processes of diagnosis and treatment are peripheral at best in Western medicine, where objective, rational, often laboratory-based, understandings place the expertise with the doctor (Cunningham and Andrews 1997).

But in asking the question what CAM is, there needs to be some idea of what dimension of therapeutic activity is being referenced. Is it a system of thinking, a group of practitioners, a practice at particular locations, a performance integrating diverse influences and so on? In the following chapters, all of these dimensions and many others will be discussed.

When CAM is mentioned, it can signify very different things for different people. For some CAM signifies pseudoscience, for others natural healing, for others an opportunity to try to deal with a chronic condition not successfully treated by biomedical approaches. It can signify a threat to biomedicine and science, or it can signify for some the duping of vulnerable people into spending large amounts of money.

So far, I have used the term 'biomedicine' to describe the dominant and most thoroughly state-legitimated therapeutic system. As with CAM terminology, there are a range of terms that have been used to capture something like the same thing. I will use a number of terms in this book that make reference to the dominant system, and in some chapters, different terms will become more prominent. The dominant form of medicine prior to the radical shifts in therapeutics in the twentieth century can be referred to as organised medicine. This simply signals that there was an occupational group of medical practitioners that had started to develop organisations that pursued the self-interest of the collective, particularly in relation to the state and to those other practitioners who they desired to exclude. Dominant therapeutic practices in many colonial states and non-western states can be referred to as Western medicine, which references all the various forms of medical practice that have been imported from Europe and North America into those states but, confusingly, would not include practices from those states that are regarded as unorthodox within their borders. Biomedicine more aptly applies to twentieth- and twenty-first-century therapeutic practices of the organised medical profession – those that have the status of medical practitioners.

Early sociological analyses of CAM emphasised the ways in which it was dominated by biomedicine. Evan Willis (1983) used case studies to illustrate different forms of dominance, for example, through subordination of occupations to medicine or limitation placed on what other professionals could practice. Gerald Larkin (1983) traced the way in which modern medicine evolved through eliminating competing healers such as herbalists and controlling emergent ones. The marginalisation of the therapeutic practices of indigenous peoples through the process of colonisation has been studied (Goldberg 1993). The growing popularity of alternative therapies since the 1960s, particularly in Anglophone countries, has been of sociological interest (Saks 2001). Reasons put forward for this rise in popularity include dissatisfaction with orthodox medicine (Sharma

1992), particularly in relation to the treatment of chronic conditions (Kelner and Wellman 1997); a growing public interest in health care generally (Northcott and Bachynsky 1993) and other trends and processes that will be discussed in Chapter 7.

In addition, exchanges of goods, services and people across the globe have taken healing practices originating in one place to a variety of other spaces, to be mixed and matched with new practices in these different spaces. There are also a host of other healing systems that flourish in their homes of origin and elsewhere. Korean migrants have brought hanbang medicine to Australia and elsewhere (Han 2000). Ayurvedic medicine from India can be found in most major Western cities, and TCM, particularly the technique of acupuncture, has a strong presence in many Western countries. This phenomenon, although being evident over millennia, has sped up over more recent decades and sparked an interest in medical diversity and medical pluralism.

Sociologists and other social scientists studying CAM can take a variety of epistemological and ontological positions. Not uncommon is an approach that appears to deny the possibility that CAM practices could have a positive biologically or physiologically based curative impact. Instead, positive effects ascribed to CAM are explained away. Similarly, the idea that people may take up CAM practices from a desire to do good for others is often not considered. To take one illustrative example, Phillip Nicholls (2001) explains away the popularity of homeopathy in nineteenth-century England by suggesting that homeopathy acted as a status symbol for patients, in that it was more refined than the gross material practices of regular medicine at that time. The idea of the status symbol is given explanatory power here. In sociology, the use of practices like acupuncture by biomedical practitioners can be viewed as an attempt by biomedicine to preserve its authority from the challenge of alternative therapies (Saks 2001). This neo-Weberian form of analysis focuses on competing interests of occupational groups, but has less to say about the experiences of those medical practitioners who opt to use alternative therapies, what I have termed deviant insiders, which are discussed in Chapter 5. Not deviant in a pejorative way, but deviant in the sense of deviating away from the norms of biomedical practice.

These neo-Weberian readings can be contrasted with some other readings. In a neo-Marxist vein, it has been suggested that people seek out CAM because their needs are not met in the technocratic world of biomedicine (Jackson and Scambler 2007). Eeva Sointu (2006: 345) takes a feminist reading of CAM patients and suggests that CAM operates on patients at the level of well-being and emotions, and that these practices can 'reach deep into the embodied and lived experiences of some of those turning to alternative and complementary medicines'. As such, Sointu focuses on 'real' effects, but not explicitly in terms of biological or physiological benefit of the actual therapy. Her focus is on an emotional fulfilment for users through engaging with CAM practices and practitioners. In line with these theoretical orientations, I will not only not make any claims about the effectiveness of CAM, but also try to avoid sociologising, psychologising or explaining away through some other means the possible effects of CAM. I will endeavour to maintain an agnostic stance on CAM efficacy.

A theme threaded throughout this book is that of medical pluralism or its variants. Medical pluralism is a concept that was coined by Charles Leslie (1976) to capture the therapeutic situation of South Asian societies, where many systems or practices of healing were available to people, such as biomedicine, traditional systems like ayurvedic medicine and folk medicines. The concept of medical pluralism has been critiqued on a number of grounds, particularly in the term failing to capture the power differentials between therapeutic systems (Penkala-Gawęcka and Rajtar 2016). The critique has led to the deployment of other terms, like medical diversity and medical landscapes (Penkala-Gawęcka and Rajtar 2016). Users of these terms suggest that they better capture the fluidity and hybridity of practices, but I am not so convinced of this. The very term 'medical' seems to reinforce the legitimacy of the dominance of biomedicine in an uncritical way. Certainly, we can think of homeopathy as homeopathic medicine, acupuncture as a branch of Chinese medicine and so on, but when the term 'medical' is used to do these other systems and practices come to mind? And it is unlikely that the term medical will bring to mind practices like spiritual healing. And should we describe prescriptions to change diet and activity as medicine? As such, I will use the term therapeutic pluralism. I am not happy with the term pluralism as for some scholars it downplays the issue of power, and I have no desire to downplay power. I, however, will use the term therapeutic pluralism throughout this book not as something that self-evidently exists, but as something that may have more or less purchase depending on a range of factors. In doing so, I will suggest that other ways of describing therapeutic diversity may be more apt in specific situations, such as using the term therapeutic hybridity to describe the healing activities inside the home.

Another caution around the use of terms like medical pluralism and therapeutic pluralism is that they may suggest that there are some coherent and closed off systems that are in operation that people can choose between. However, drawing on Volker Scheid's (2002) argument, it is important to note that all therapeutic systems, including biomedicine and traditional medical systems like ayurveda and Chinese medicine, are dynamic, fluid and changeable, as are the ways in which people use these therapeutic approaches. In their fluidity and dynamism, different systems will take in aspects of other therapeutic approaches and remould them in doing so. This is not just when biomedicine takes on board other therapeutic modalities, such as acupuncture discussed in Chapter 5, but also traditional therapeutic approaches using biomedical concepts or techniques. This further complicates those definitional issues around what is orthodox and what is alternative.

In this book, I will be considering the how and the where of therapeutic pluralism. Where can we see it more likely to operate, or have more opportunities to operate, and where is medical hegemony likely to be more evident. I will argue, for example, that therapeutic pluralism is more or less available at the level of the household, the level of the clinic and the practitioner, the level of the professional organisation and the level of the state and its regulations, and indeed at the level of something broader and more ephemeral, that of the culture of a society. Throughout, the concept of therapeutic pluralism will be problematised, and it will be considered in connection with statist medicine. Statist medicine references the multiple ways in which therapeutic practices are both supported by and entangled in the state and its institutions. The state plays a central role in promoting, allowing or constraining therapeutic pluralism.

Some authors suggest that rather than talk of medical systems, such as biomedicine, ayurveda and so on, it is more useful to talk of medical practices (Ranganathan 2018). Medical systems imply that a system is homogenous and systematised. Many authors contest that there is such a level of standardisation (see Scheid 2002) and that to consider medical systems in this way suggests dichotomies and oppositions that might not be so clear in practice. People, in their health-seeking practices, can forge together what health professionals may see as contradictory and incompatible systems, such as religious practices and institutional medical practices in India (Ranganathan 2018). So, a focus on practices can help us to consider the complexities, overlaps, incoherences and so on within and between these 'named' systems. The possibilities for pluralism are further boosted by the instability of concepts like the medical (Roy and Attewell 2018) and its contrasts such as alternative medicine. As stated, the object called CAM, or any of its variants, is not stable over time or place, and could appear along a continuum from subaltern or folk-healing practices through to orthodox hospital-based practices. We need then to consider the relationship between therapeutic practices in their specificity and be wary of generalising from particular instances to statements about that relationship.

From a sociological perspective, another important dimension of demarcation emerges that is associated with professional occupations. At this level, the practice or the system is not so crucial as the political manoeuvring of different associations to control therapeutic markets. The medical profession has been most successful at this occupational strategy, being able to exercise occupational closure by excluding those not medically qualified from calling themselves doctors or medical practitioners. In this sense, systems and practices can drastically change. The therapeutic system and practices of the mid-nineteenth century when occupational closure was first enacted are markedly different from the systems and practices of the early twenty-first century. What has remained is the power of particular elites within medicine to determine what practices are legitimated and what ones are disempowered, as will be outlined in Chapter 2.

This book does not try to settle the dispute about the reasons for interest in CAM but does provide insights into the relationship between CAM and orthodox medicine in contemporary times. As Philip Tovey et al. (2004) state, 'To understand the contemporary forms and contents of CAM there is a need to step back from the often hurriedly established demands of policy-makers, and to explicitly include in analyses reference to how the arena is marked by complexity and contingency, diversity and dispute and is in a state of constant change'.

The chapters in this book explore some of the many different manifestations of therapeutic pluralism. In Chapter 2, the focus is on the efforts of professional organisations to limit therapeutic pluralism, achieved in large part through gaining legitimisation by the state and the capacity, or not, to regulate what other practitioners could do and claim. This chapter examines the way in which orthodox and unorthodox, regular and irregular, conventional and unconventional, and mainstream and alternative practices were established, particularly in the Western world. Chapter 3 goes on to consider ways in which the disciplining of what has become biomedicine impacts on the disciplining and the credibility of non-biomedical approaches. It also looks at efforts to connect up therapeutic practices into integrated approaches, suggesting that these efforts are undertaken on the terms of the dominant therapeutic practice. The increasing interest and deployment of indigenous healing practices are also noted, and this development raises a different set of possibilities around therapeutic pluralism.

The next three chapters explore specific modalities in different settings, and the way they too are disciplined or transformative. Chapter 4 provides an in-depth look at the efforts of one modality, chiropractic, a therapeutic approach born in the United States, to gain some of the prestige, status and resources of biomedicine. If it was completely successful, it could be argued that an enhanced form of therapeutic pluralism at state level is obtained. However, in this chapter, I suggest that the gains made by chiropractic to gain state resources come with costs, one cost being the limitation of its therapeutic claims. Chapter 5 looks at a therapeutic modality that has gained some popularity in the West although it has its origins in China, TCM and particularly acupuncture. Here again, we see some success in the uptake of Chinese medicine both in China and in the West, but in finding a place in the therapeutic marketplace the modality transforms, and arguably, transforms some of the other modalities including biomedicine, that it intersects with. This chapter, and the following one on therapeutic practices in the Indian subcontinent, indicates the important role of broader social, economic and political trends that can support or challenge therapeutic pluralism. In countries that have been colonised, like India, therapeutic practices based in tradition can become entwined with nationalistic and anti-colonial concerns. However, in addition to these major systems of therapeutics in such countries, such as biomedicine, ayurvedic medicine and siddha medicine, there exists a range of therapeutic activities that are not overseen by the state and thrive in undisciplined forms – the subaltern therapeutic practices.

Chapter 7 shifts the focus to individuals, citizens and people deploying different health practices and approaches. At this level, in people's homes, therapeutic pluralism can perhaps be most clearly seen. All homes are different; there are no standardised practices and therapeutic activity is undisciplined. In Chapter 7, what happens when these unruly domestic practices enter the clinical consultation is also documented. The following chapter on the use of CAM in the face of cancer brings to the fore the high stakes that can be at play when CAM use and life-threatening illness come into contact. Forms of disciplining go hand in hand with pluralistic practices as the imperatives to pursue health in the face of possible death can come up against the limitations of biomedicine.

In exploring these quite different spaces and places of therapeutic activity, the tension between discipline, standardisation and orthodoxy on the one side, and autonomy, diversity and plurality on the other, come to the fore. CAM, like biomedicine, is anything but static, and the relationship between therapeutic practices is ever evolving and dynamic, full of friction and full of possibilities.

References

Cunningham, A. and Andrews, B. (1997) Introduction: Western medicine as contested knowledge, in A. Cunningham and B. Andrews (eds.), *Western medicine as contested knowledge*, Manchester and New York: Manchester University Press, pp. 1–23.

Goldberg, D. (1993) *Imperial medicine and indigenous societies*, Manchester: Manchester University Press.

Han, G.S. (2000) *Health and medicine under capitalism: Korean migrants in Australia*, Cranbury, NJ: Associated University Presses.

Herzlich, C. (2001) Patients, practitioners, social scientists and the multiple logics of caring and healing, in R. Jütte, M. Eklöf and M. Nelson (eds.), *Historical aspects of unconventional medicine: Approaches, concepts and case studies*, Sheffield: European Association for the History of Medicine and Health Publications, pp. 27–35.

Jackson, S. and Scambler, G. (2007) Perceptions of evidence-based medicine: Traditional acupuncturists in the UK and resistance to biomedical modes of evaluation. *Sociology of Health & Illness*, 29, 3, 412–429.

Jütte, R. (2001) Alternative medicine and medico-historical semantics, in R. Jütte, M. Eklöf and M. Nelson (eds.), *Historical aspects of unconventional medicine: Approaches, concepts, case studies*, Sheffield: European Association for the History of Medicine and Health Publications, pp. 11–26.

Kelner, M. and Wellman, B. (1997) Health care and consumer choice: Medical and alternative therapies, *Social Science & Medicine*, 45, 2, 203–212.

Larkin, G. (1983) *Occupational monopoly and modern medicine*, London: Tavistock Press.

Leslie, C. (1976) *Asian medical systems: A comparative study*. Berkeley: University of California Press.

National Center for Complementary and Alternative Medicine (2000) *Expanding horizons of healthcare: Five-year strategic plan 2001–2005*, https://nccih.nih.gov/sites/nccam.nih.gov/files/about/plans/fiveyear/fiveyear.pdf accessed 18 October 2019.

Nicholls, P. (2001) The social construction and organisation of medical marginality: The case of homeopathy in mid nineteenth century Britain, in R. Jütte, M. Eklöf and M. Nelson (eds.), *Historical aspects of unconventional medicine: Approaches, concepts and case studies*, Sheffield: European Association for the History of Medicine and Health Publications, pp. 163–181.

Northcott, H. and Bachynsky, J. (1993) Concurrent utilization of chiropractic, prescription medicines, nonprescription medicine and alternative health care, *Social Science & Medicine*, 37, 3, 431–435.

Ohnuki-Tierney, E. (1997) The reduction of personhood to brain and rationality? Japanese contestation of medical high technology, in A. Cunningham and B. Andrews (eds.), *Western medicine as contested knowledge*, Manchester and New York: Manchester University Press, pp. 212–240.

Penkala-Gawęcka, D. and Rajtar, M. (2016) Introduction to the special issue 'medical pluralism and beyond', *Anthropology & Medicine*, 23, 2, 129–134.

Pokladnikova, J. and Telec, I. (2020) Provision of complementary and alternative medicine: Compliance with the health professional requirements, *Health Policy*, 124, 3, 311–316.

Ranganathan, S. (2018) Re-thinking the 'medical' through the lens of the 'indigenous': Narratives from Mahanubhav healing shrines in Maharashtra, India, in R.D. Roy and G.N.A. Attewell (eds.), *Locating the medical*, Oxford: Oxford University Press, pp. 219–234.

Roberts, C.S., Baker, F., Hann, D., Runfola, J., Witt, C., McDonald, J., Livingston, M.L., Ruiterman, J., Ampela, R., Kaw, O.C. and Blanchard, C. (2006) Patient-physician communication regarding use of complementary therapies during cancer treatment, *Journal of Psychosocial Oncology*, 23, 4, 35–60.

Roy, R.D. and Attewell, G.N.A. (2018) Introduction: Locating the medical, in R.D. Roy and G.N.A. Attewell (eds.), *Locating the medical*, Oxford: Oxford University Press, pp. 1–20.

Saks, M. (2001) Alternative medicine and the health care division of labour: Present trends and future prospects, *Current Sociology*, 49, 3, 119–134.

Scheid, V. (2002) *Chinese medicine in contemporary China: Plurality and synthesis*, Durham, NC: Duke University Press.

Sharma, S. (1992) *Complementary medicine today: Practitioners and patients*, London: Routledge.

Sointu, E. (2006) The search for wellbeing in alternative and complementary health practices, *Sociology of Health & Illness*, 28, 330–349.

Tovey, P., Easthope, G. and Adams, J. (2004) Introduction, in P. Tovey, G. Easthope and J. Adams (eds.), *The mainstreaming of complementary and alternative medicine: Studies in social context*, London and New York: Routledge, pp. 1–7.

Willis, E. (1983) *Medical dominance: The division of labour in Australian healthcare*, Sydney: George Allen & Unwin.

2

STATE MEDICINE, REGULATING PRACTICES AND THE CREATION OF ALTERNATIVES

The history of 'quackery' and the regulation of medicine at a time when organised medicine had little therapeutic value to offer are considered. The creation of alternatives is an outcome of these processes. The development of biomedicine increasingly takes the patient's input out of the diagnostic picture as laboratory medicine and technological development reframe diagnosis. Despite these developments, orthodox medical practitioners continue to be interested in CAM therapeutics.

Efforts to limit therapeutic pluralism evolve as the occupational groupings of medical practitioners professionalise and, through state legitimation, can exclude others from gaining the credibility and status of a medical practitioner or doctor. The outcome of this relationship in Anglophone regions like Britain, Australasia and North America was not to foster therapeutic pluralism but, rather, establish a therapeutic hegemony. In achieving state legitimation, the medical profession then played a central role in determining what is 'alternative' medicine, that is, those practices that are not given credibility by the medical profession. But it is of course not so simple, as some practices might be alternative in many jurisdictions but are given state support in others. So the term 'statist medicine' is a useful one here to indicate that there are practices that are given status by the state through regulation or other forms of support for those who undertake the practices, but those practices do not sit comfortably within a notion of orthodox medical practice. The case of homeopathy, particularly in the United Kingdom, illustrates this well and will be discussed in this chapter.

The notion of alternative medicine can only gain purchase once orthodox medicine has gained some stability (Bivins 2007), a stability that is achieved through its relationship with the state. Statist medicine refers to both the practices of conventional medicine or biomedicine and the state regulatory apparatus in which it is embedded, including the legal requirements around diagnosis, prescription, medical claims-making, market approval and state subsidisation of medicines (Dew and Armstrong n.d.). Statist medicine is an outcome of a complex interplay of the interests of the medical profession to exclude therapeutic rivals, the functional needs of the state and the impact of commercial interests, particularly of pharmaceutical companies (Abbott 1988; Dew 2003; Larkin 1983; Willis 1983).

In the latter half of the twentieth century, the dominant position of biomedicine came under challenge from, among other things, CAM (Broom et al. 2014). A common critique is that CAM therapies have not been adequately tested and so neither medical practitioners nor patients should use them, and some should be banned altogether (Ernst and Smith 2018). Yet the medical profession itself gained its prestige, privileges and social status when the treatments used, such as bloodletting and the use of mercury, would be seen as barbarous today. Many medical practitioners today use a range of therapies which include what some regard as unorthodox or alternative. This chapter explores these apparent paradoxes by providing an overview of the development of the established medical profession and looks at the popularity and proliferation of alternative therapeutic practices. By looking at these developments, we can better understand the relationship between regulation, discipline, the validation of medical knowledge and the therapeutic possibilities that are available. This discussion highlights the tension between the desire to regulate and control therapeutic practices on the one hand, and the support for unorthodox therapeutic practices outside state and medical control on the other.

Controlling practices

Efforts at establishing boundaries between credible and discreditable therapeutic practices and therapists have been made for millennia. A dominating therapeutic tradition will attempt to expel heretics from within its ranks and discredit quacks outside its ranks. Akin to a religious heretic, a medical heretic can be described as someone within the orthodox medical establishment who uses a therapy that is not accepted medical practice. Concerns about medical heretics have existed since ancient times in Western medicine. Galen of Pergamon (129AD to C216) is arguably the central figure in the development of the Western medical tradition, and he called his opponents 'charlatans, quacks and medical murderers' (Nutton 1995b: 58), terminology that has a familiar ring today.

In the medieval period, those who practised unconventional therapeutic methods could run great risks. Five 'sorcerers' were burnt at the stake in 1403 for failing to cure the madness of the French king Charles VI (Nutton 1995a). There were, however, less dramatic attempts to regulate the market by national, ecclesiastical, university and local authorities. Medieval attempts to facilitate medical hegemony and undermine therapeutic pluralism lay in the guild system. Guilds thrived during this time, and they were able to limit the number of people who could practise a particular occupation. But 'patient preference for a bonesetter, herbalist or wise-woman could defy even a tight guild-based system' (Nutton 1995a: 168). The lack of monopoly by any one group of medical practitioners continued into the seventeenth century in Europe, so that people had greater independence in deciding who to see (Wear 1995).

An increasingly important way of controlling therapeutic practices was by legal means, or in earlier times, royal decrees. However, attempts to limit who can practice therapeutics could be challenged by the constraints on states to provide health services for its population. Denmark introduced a Quackery Law in 1794 that allowed for the imprisonment or fining of those who practiced medicine without a license. However, due to a lack of doctors and the presence of skilled folk healers, there was a reluctance to enforce such a law (Bonderup 2001). Quackery laws could however be enforced if the healer was threatening the income of the licensed practitioners (Ling 2001).

There were counterposing laws to quackery prevention laws in many European countries. In 1873, a law was introduced throughout the German empire that allowed anyone to provide medical treatment for a fee (Stolberg 2001). The desire to allow unlicensed practitioners to operate in sparsely populated and under-served areas in Sweden led to an Authorisation to Practise the Art of Doctoring Act in 1915, where the medical profession lost its monopoly until this Act was abolished in 1960 (Eklöf 2001). The 1960 Act shifted the language from the art of doctoring to physicians who practice the profession of medicine, so that from that time a clear boundary could be drawn between qualified doctors, who were the only ones who now could call themselves doctors. These examples of legislation in different jurisdictions are suggestive of the complex relationship between the state and therapeutic groups or occupations that is replete with tensions and contradictory tendencies.

In colonial settler societies, where Europeans have colonised other nations, such as in America, Australia and New Zealand, the regulation of therapeutic practices has included the regulation, or suppression, of indigenous health practices. Settlers and colonisers could actively suppress or discourage the health practices of indigenous peoples. In New Zealand, a Tohunga Suppression Act of 1907 restricted the rights of Māori to go to a traditional Māori healer, the Tohunga. Tohunga were specialists in healthcare practices, and with the passing of the Act, they could be imprisoned if they continued to practice (Belgrave 1985). The Act was established, in part, to direct Māori towards Western systems of treatment. This was despite the fact that most Māori were living in rural areas with very poor access to Western medical facilities, and that hospital boards were reluctant to admit Māori patients (Lange 1999). This led to the loss of indigenous systems of knowledge in a range of areas, including childbirth practices (Kenney 2011). The Act was not repealed until 1962. In other countries, cultural traditions were banned for allegedly health reasons. In Canada, ceremonial gatherings like the potlatch and the sun dance were at one time banned for fear of spreading tuberculosis (Kelm 2010).

Creating alternatives

Phillip Nicholls argues that we should consider the process of one group of practitioners excluding another group as a cause of therapeutic difference, rather than exclusion being a result of therapeutic difference (Nicholls 2001). He illustrates this using the example of homeopathy in nineteenth-century England. As a therapeutic approach, homeopathy was in stark contrast to the regular medical therapeutics of the nineteenth century. The founder of homeopathy, Samuel Hahnemann (1755–1843) identified three principles of the approach, the law of similars, the law of infinitesimals and the use of a single remedy. The law of similars states that substances that produce symptoms in a healthy person would relieve those symptoms in those who suffer from them. The law of infinitesimals is the potency of a substance increases as it is diluted and refined (Bivins 2007). This is based on a view that the refined substance affects the vital spirit, and so is not working with the physiological mechanisms invoked by a materialist medical approach. The substance to be used was diluted and succussed or shaken to enable it to acquire the ability to affect the vital spirit. Hahnemann coined the term 'allopathy' to describe orthodox practitioners. Allopathy attempts to remove or oppose disease causes and suppress or palliate symptoms (Nicholls 1988: 3).

In nineteenth-century England, prominent homeopaths who were medically trained saw themselves as part of the medical profession but were drawing on homeopathy to reform it. The desire to reform medicine was driven in part by concerns about its therapeutic approaches, including the influence of heroic medicine, which will be discussed in the next section. In contrast, 'orthodox' practitioners, such as the members of Provincial Medical and Surgical Association, embarked on processes to try to exclude or marginalise homeopaths in their ranks, such as making it unethical for members to professionally consort with homeopaths. Homeopaths were then compelled to form their own organisations, so reinforcing schisms that had not until then been so apparent (Nicholls 2001). With the opprobrium of the regular practitioners, organisations like the British Homeopathic Society became more popular. Besides adhering to understandings of healing that were now untenable to a developing (but as yet therapeutically ineffective) medical science, medical homeopaths also betrayed the profession of medicine by providing mothers and homemakers with expertise over the use of their medications. They did this through the use of customised medicine chests and the availability of popular books, such as *Homeopathic Domestic Medicine*, that fostered self-diagnosis and treatment in the home (Nicholls 2001). Having children treated in the home meant lost fees for regular practitioners.

Homeopathy flourished in many countries including Germany, France and the United States, and in the latter, it was particularly suited to a geographically dispersed population in a social climate that rejected elitism (Bivins 2007). Homeopathy appealed to both well-heeled fee-paying clients and to the rural poor, the latter being serviced through the purchase of homeopathic kits that allowed for the self-administration of remedies. In many countries in Europe, homeopathy provided a challenge to organised medicine in the nineteenth century. In Bavaria, it became a major challenge from the 1830s and stalwarts of the medical profession took it up, and it was taught in medical training (Stolberg 2001). However, its popularity was relatively short-lived, going into decline well before the end of the nineteenth century (Stolberg 2001). Even where the practice of homeopathy was illegal, popular support could allow it to thrive. In Iceland in the late 1800s, when homeopaths were not allowed to practice medicine, one person practicing homeopathy was acquitted by a judge, who had been a patient of that practitioner in the previous year (Pétursdóttir 2001).

In the British context, homeopathy could retain a relatively strong foothold due to its patronage by royalty and the wealthy. In the mid-1800s, the London Homeopathic Hospital included the following as patrons: 'Her Royal Highness the Duchess of Cambridge, His Grace the Duke of Beaufort, Field Marshall the Marquis of Worcester, the Earl of Essex, Viscount Sydney, Lord Gray, Viscount Maldon, Lord Francis Gordon' (Nicholls 2001: 172). In other countries, such as in Portugal, where homeopathy was patronised by members of the aristocracy in the late nineteenth century, it was later to gain no purchase in the healthcare system and was successfully positioned by the medical establishment as a 'fallacious' and 'sinister' practice (Almeida 2012).

Regulation by the state

Before medical regulation in Britain, a range of community-based healers provided health care. The 'orthodox' medical occupations themselves were divided into three broad categories. Physicians were the elite of British medicine, being university trained and mixing with other social elites. Surgeons were the craftsmen, a less prestigious manual occupational grouping. Apothecaries had a lower status still due to their connection with trade, selling their merchandise of herbal preparations and other remedies (Nicholls 1988). Modern medicine evolved through eliminating what Gerald Larkin calls itinerant and community-based healers and controlling emergent ones (Larkin 1983).

The occupational distinctions between physicians, surgeons and apothecaries had become increasingly irrelevant as these practitioners had more in common with each than they did with the elitist London colleges which maintained these demarcations (Nicholls 1988), hence the term general practitioner (GP) came to dominate the titles used by these groups. The merging of apothecaries, surgeons and physicians in nineteenth-century England was an early development in the professionalisation of medicine (Abbott 1988), and with this greater level of unity, the profession could undertake the intense legislative lobbying that would eventually lead to the passing of the 1858 Medical Act (Waddington 1977). Prior to the passing of the 1858 Act, the concept of a qualified or registered practitioner had no place in English law (Waddington 1977). The Act gave the General

Medical Council powers to control who could practice medicine by establishing a system of medical registration. Although not restricting the practice of medicine to doctors, the General Medical Council established by the Act was so powerful that it could veto other occupations' claims for recognition (Larkin 1983). Subsequently, healthcare occupations such as nurses and physiotherapists have had to seek medical patronage in the same ways as the medical profession had previously sought state patronage (Larkin 1983). The medical profession was now effectively organised and its relationship with the state allowed it to exert control over the growing healthcare division of labour.

The 1858 Act in the United Kingdom was not, however, an outright victory for the regular medical practitioners of the day. As noted, at this time homoeopathy was very popular and posed a serious challenge to orthodox medicine. Because of the power of homeopathy, a clause was inserted into legislation that would ensure that homoeopaths could practise. The effect of this right to practise has meant that homoeopathy has maintained a place in regulated medical practice in the United Kingdom, though a rather vulnerable place. In England, for example, homoeopathic physicians enjoyed royal patronage and were licensed to practice under the National Health Service. Although a medical orthodoxy dominated in Britain, the existence of a medical homeopathy allowed for a partial form of therapeutic pluralism. There was at least some clearly demarcated alternative officially sanctioned.

Apart from the homoeopaths, the 1858 Medical Act had a dramatic impact in excluding other therapeutic practices, now created and identified as alternative, unorthodox or irregular. In Britain, it took another 135 years before alternative therapies were able to gain recognition and favourable legislation as separate occupational groups. This occurred with the passing of the Osteopaths Act 1993 in the United Kingdom (Fisher and Ward 1994). In the United States, licensing laws took a lot longer to take effect than in the United Kingdom with apprenticeship systems the common route to medical practice until the late 1800s.

It might be thought that orthodox medicine gained its foothold in statist medicine, obtaining state regulation along with high status due to its therapeutic practices being based in science and having the credibility of scientific practices. But the occupation of medicine became professionalised during the age of heroic medicine and gained state privileges as well as the exclusion of rival, now alternative, therapies from such special consideration at this time. The age of heroic medicine affected Europe and its colonies and was particularly prominent in the United States between the 1780s and the 1850s. Medical treatment during this period included bloodletting, administration of large doses of calomel (mercurous chloride) and other dangerous mineral drugs, purgatives, emetics and venesection (Coulter 1973; Kaufman 1971). The approach of heroic medicine can be summed up as a process of bloodletting, purging and puking. This form of treatment was based on the theory of humours where, for example, fever was caused by miasmas or noxious substances arising from filth and putrefying matter that corrupted the natural humours of the body. Treatment was aimed at driving out the vitiated humours (Duffy 1979). And this driving out could take drastic forms.

An influential exponent of this style of heroic medicine was Benjamin Rush, who, in the early 1800s, was considered the greatest physician of his day (Duffy 1979). He had great kudos, having been a signatory to the Declaration of Independence, and he had served as Surgeon General for the American Continental Army. For Rush, disease resulted from 'capillary tension' and the only cure for this was bloodletting and purging. In his quest for cure, it is alleged that Rush 'was willing to remove up to four-fifths of the blood in the body' (Kaufman 1971: 2). Rush was about as far removed from natural healing as one could be and believed that one of the hindrances to the development of medicine was the reliance on the powers of nature to cure disease (Duffy 1979).

For Rush, desperate diseases required desperate remedies. The common practice was to bleed to syncope or unconsciousness, and then on recovery, the patient was bled again. General bloodletting was carried out by venesection, and local bloodletting by the use of leeches. Blistering was also a treatment of choice, where a second-degree burn would be created, and would become infected and suppurate. The pus was seen as a sign of the infection being drawn out of the system (Kaufman 1971). Purging was carried out using emetics to induce vomiting, and cathartics to evacuate the bowels. Calomel, which is mercurous chloride, was also given in large doses for a variety of conditions. These massive doses produced salivation, loosening of the teeth, falling out of the hair and other symptoms of acute mercury poisoning. As calomel would also irritate the bowel, it was sometimes given with opium. Benjamin Rush attended to George Washington, most probably hastening his death. Washington's treatment included repeated bleedings, repeated blistering and repeated doses of calomel (Bivins 2007).

Surgery also came with great risks throughout the nineteenth and early twentieth century during the times of state recognition of the medical profession. The patient receiving surgery was likely to be drunk in order to numb the pain. The surgeon would have hands and instruments that were not sterile and was likely to have the blood of previous patients on his frock with no understanding at the time of the need for hygiene (Sigsworth 1972: 109). Although Eric Sigsworth suggests that this picture of surgery in the nineteenth century may be overstated, the surgical mortality rate was as high as seventeen percent in some hospitals (Sigsworth 1972).

Alternatives to orthodox medicine in the nineteenth century were not necessarily a more comforting option. The following quote is taken from a work by Sebastian Kneipp, regarded as a nineteenth-century pioneer of natural healing. He was particularly devoted to the water cure, or what today we would call hydrotherapy. One water cure technique was the affusion, where cold water would be poured over the body. Of affusions, Kneipp says

> Invalids and weak persons seldom stand the shock of the first affusion, and to no beginner is the sensation a pleasant one. I have seen strong men, who

> beforehand had treated the idea with derision, turn pale and tremble like aspen-leaves in vain endeavour to disguise the pain occasioned by the cold-water gush. This potent effect speaks volumes in favour of its invigorating and bracing effects.
>
> *(Kneipp (1893[1979]): 47)*

Although these approaches to healing challenge our contemporary understandings of therapeutics, the average patient of the day might insist on receiving such treatments (Kaufman 1971). Within the worldview of the time, the materia medica of heroic medicine worked. It worked because it produced

> visible and predictable physiological effects: purges purged, emetics induced vomiting, opium soothed pain and moderated diarrhoea. Bleeding, too, seemed obviously to alter the body's internal balance, as evidenced both by a changed pulse and the very quantity of blood drawn.
>
> *Rosenberg 1992: 15*

For the patient, these reactions to the poisons were clear signs that the body was ridding itself of disease. With this worldview, mercury was the most flexible drug because of its obvious manifestations and power. Other poisons, like arsenic and strychnine, were also used because of the strong responses that they produced. Drugs had to produce (or exhibit) perceptible physiological effects that could be witnessed by both the physician and the patient.

But the decline of heroic medicine did not lead to anything recognisably therapeutic by today's standards. When the use of bloodletting and purging started to fall from favour, opiates, narcotics and alcohol became the therapies of choice (Kaufman 1971: 112). Between the 1850s and 1870s in the United States, there developed an increasing emphasis on diet and regimen among regular physicians, as well as the use of alcoholic beverages as stimulants (Rosenberg 1992: 26). Regimen refers to a planned way of living that can include diet, exercise and consumption of medicines (Bivins 2007).

The remnants of heroic medicine could be seen into the twentieth century, with the lancet still being used in the 1930s. It was through this period of heroic medicine that orthodox medicine became organised, politicised and gained access to state benefits. The medical profession was able to control hospitals that received state funding and also secured state grants for their educational establishments. Medical professionals also acquired the benefits of being expert witnesses in court cases, certifying causes of death and so on. Practitioners of alternative therapies were excluded from acquiring those benefits.

Laboratory medicine and medical devices

Medicine changed dramatically in the latter part of the nineteenth century and in the twentieth century. An important element in what would increasingly be called biomedicine was the central role that was taken up by the laboratory. In the mid-nineteenth century, the Paris Clinical School became an influential centre (Rosenberg 1987). It has been argued by Michel Foucault (2003) that at this time the specific form of practice that constitutes modern medicine emerged. For Foucault, the mechanism of this change in medicine is found in the 'gaze': there was a transformation in the way doctors 'saw' the objects of their science that brought about a radical change in the practice of medicine. There was a switch from a medicine of health to a medicine of normality. The doctor now defined standards of an ideal physical state and did not simply attempt to restore the body to a non-diseased state. Prior to this change of gaze, disease had been seen as a general physiological state, an imbalance in, or a corruption of, the humours, not a result of specific agents with predictable patterns (Rosenberg 1987). Now disease was to be perceived as a visible entity, a germ or a specific lesion, which could be measured. Disease left traces in the body, specific lesions for specific diseases. The microscope and chemical testing were incorporated into the diagnostic process, identifying those traces in the body. Hospitals were now settings where the symptoms could be correlated with the findings of autopsies (Rosenberg 1987).

Before the invention of stethoscopes, electrocardiograms, laboratory diagnosis and the many diagnostic instruments that exist today, patients would have available to them the same signs of the condition they were suffering from as the doctor had. Doctors would be led to their diagnosis by asking patients questions, and looking at such physical signs as skin colour, the colour of the palate, and the colour, smell and taste of urine. But with the invention of the stethoscope, which was commercially produced in the 1850s, the doctor had available to him (or more rarely her) an instrument that delivered signs (sounds from the chest) that were not available to the patient. Now the doctor could diagnose on the basis of the unseen. The stethoscope, the laboratory test and later the capacity to see inside the body with radiography and other developments meant that from this point on, doctors could exercise more control over information than the patients and could decide whether to make information available to patients or not. The power of the patient declined as the medical profession came to dominate the use of medical technologies. Some argue that we will see this control of information by the medical profession undermined in an age of the Internet. Ready access to information, opinions and perspectives on different diseases, their causation and treatment can enter into the decision-making processes for patients, as we will see in Chapter 7.

Challenge of alternative medicine

Despite regulation of medical practices, alternative medicine has always found support both within and outside the regulated medical profession. At various times, homoeopathy, acupuncture, chiropractic and osteopathy have had strong support in English-speaking and other countries. As noted, homoeopathy, in particular, posed a threat to the orthodox medicine of the time in the nineteenth century, gaining fashionable status and community support in Britain (Nicholls 1988), Australia (Willis 1983), the United States (Coulter 1984; Kaufman 1971) and New Zealand (Dew 2003).

Homoeopathy posed such a challenge to orthodox medicine of the time because many highly educated and orthodox practitioners abandoned regular medicine and took up homoeopathy. In the United States, homoeopaths were generally receiving higher fees for their services and had more successful practices than their orthodox colleagues, and it is estimated that ten percent of medical practitioners practised homoeopathy at the beginning of the twentieth century (Berliner 1984). Homoeopaths established the first national medical organisation in the United States, the American Institute of Homoeopathy, to regulate its members and ensure standards of education. Orthodox histories make the claim that homoeopathy was really a treatment which let nature take its course and proved that this method was better than heroic medicine, therefore playing a useful part in the decline of heroic medicine (Bivins 2007; Coulter 1973).

In early nineteenth-century America, issues between orthodox and unorthodox medicine came to be defined by regular physicians as 'science versus quackery', with irregular physicians posing a threat to an innocent public. Irregulars, who had licenses to practice medicine but were not part of the orthodox medical profession, such as homoeopaths and those who used botanical medicine, defined the relationship as free competition versus monopoly, and that people should be free to make their own healthcare choices (Starr 1982: 58).

In nineteenth-century America, there were thousands of homoeopathic practitioners, and homoeopaths had the same legal status as allopaths, or the orthodox medical practitioners of the time, and eclectics (Coulter 1984). Eclectics combined the use of allopathy and homeopathy, to the chagrin of both groups, but rejected the use of bloodletting and relied on botanical drugs (Duffy 1979; Rothstein 1988). But in the early twentieth century, homeopathy went into decline. This phenomenon of decline resulted from complex cultural and social processes, though opponents of homeopathy have claimed that the decline was due to the triumph of scientific medicine. For example, medical apologists claimed that the discovery of sulphonamides in 1935 foreshadowed the demise of homoeopathy (Beaven 1989). Sulphonamides, in this argument, are considered to be the first recognised pharmaceutical treatment of the modern pharmacopoeia. Accounts along these lines fail to recognise that the decline of homoeopathy occurred before medicine had much in the way of therapeutic capability that would be regarded by contemporary standards as effective. Homoeopathy was well in decline before the discovery of sulphonamides. Cultural changes in the perception of science and technology, changes in the therapeutic relationship with moves to hospital-based medicine and shorter consultation times, and the weakening of homoeopathy due to internal struggles, all played a part in the decline of homoeopathy (Kaufman 1971).

An important element in the decline of homeopathy in the United States was the impact of the 1910 Flexner Report on medical education. The standards set following the report, including laboratory teaching, meant the demise of many medical schools, particularly affecting homeopathic ones. In 1900, there were 22 homeopathy schools in the United States but by 1923 there were only two (Kaufman 1971), although one homeopathic hospital in Pennsylvania survived into the 1950s (Bivins 2007).

A different explanation of homeopathy's decline is offered by Nicholls (1988), who argues that homeopathy did not resonate with the requirements of a capitalist society. There were several reasons for this. Homeopathy stressed the unique features of each patient, and the longer consultations required to explore these features clashed with requirements for high patient turnover. The concept of identifying a specific remedy for each individual clashed with the pharmaceutical goals of developing universal remedies that have the potential for great profits.

As already noted, homoeopathy still maintains a strong presence in statist medicine in England with medically trained homeopathic doctors integrated into the National Health Service when it was established, although in 1950 homeopathic training was denied public funding (Bivins 2007). In more recent times, many integrated medical service centres in the National Health Service offer homeopathy (Sharp et al. 2018). In tension with this is the 2018 announcement of the withdrawal of National Health Service funding for homeopathic remedies in some hospitals where it was previously funded.

Homeopathy is also practised in many other nations, but is particularly strong in Sri Lanka, Pakistan and India (Coulter 1984). Different political regimes could allow for greater or lesser incorporation of CAM practices. Prior to the Russian revolution, homeopathy was given a boost in Russia because of support from the Russian Orthodox Church. Homeopathy then suffered for this association post-revolution (Dinges 2001). From the 1970s, in the postcolonial countries of India and Brazil, homeopathy became integrated into the public health system and treatment was covered by national health insurance schemes (Dinges 2001). Switzerland, in 2017, incorporated a number of CAM specialities in its public health insurance system, and support for CAM is embedded in that country's constitution (Pokladnikova and Telec 2020). Not far from Switzerland, in Spain, on the other hand, all of its main political parties have opposed any support of CAM (Cano-Orón 2019).

Other popular modalities in English-speaking countries include osteopathy and chiropractic. By the end of the nineteenth century, bonesetters, one of the precursors to osteopaths and chiropractors, flourished in Britain (Willis 1983). However, as noted earlier, it would take until 1993 before osteopaths gained state regulation in the United Kingdom, and that regulation limited their scope of practice. In Australia, chiropractors, osteopaths and TCM practitioners have protected titles (Brosnan 2015).

The case of osteopaths took a very different trajectory in the United States than it did in the United Kingdom. In the United States, A.T. Still founded osteopathy in the late nineteenth century. Osteopathy originally viewed disease as an effect of anatomic displacement, particularly of spinal vertebrae. In the United States, osteopathy very quickly abandoned its precepts and adopted drug-based medicine. By the 1950s, osteopaths began to be accepted as physicians by medical practitioners' organisations, and by 1960, there were 38 states where doctors of osteopathic medicine were eligible for unlimited licensure and so had the same scope of practice as medical doctors (Gevitz 1988). In 1967, the American Medical Association's House of Delegates was authorised to negotiate the conversion of schools of osteopathy to orthodox colleges. By 1988, osteopathy had 15 accredited schools, maintained 175 recognised hospitals, had over 25,000 licensed physicians and surgeons, published its own journals and provided health care for up to 25 million Americans. Outside of the United States, osteopathy has not been granted the same privileges as the medical profession. Osteopathy may then be practiced in quite different ways depending, in part, on the profession's relationship to state regulation. Chiropractic, which will be focused on in Chapter 4, has not achieved the same privileges inside the United States as osteopathy, or anywhere else.

It is evident then that the relationship between orthodox medical practice and CAM practices varies from country to country, and the examples of homoeopathy and osteopathy noted here are simply illustrative of arrangements in particular jurisdictions. CAM practitioners can work as medical practitioners, as with doctors of osteopathy in the United States and medical homoeopaths in the United Kingdom, or they can have their own associations that regulate its practices within a more limited scope of practice, as with osteopaths in the United Kingdom, or they can have no specific state regulation, as with many therapists throughout the world.

CAM inside the boundaries of orthodox medicine

Orthodox medicine's response to the popularity of alternative therapies ranges from 'extreme scepticism about the scientificity of anything lying outside its boundaries to attempted incorporation of some of the techniques of alternative practitioners into its own sphere of work' (Kelleher 1994: xv). The danger of following the latter course is that if the profession incorporates alternative practices it may lessen to some extent the basis of conventional medicine's cultural authority. This is the balancing act, which the boundary maintainers of the medical profession must perform. This balancing act will be explored further in the following chapters.

A number of studies in Britain indicate a high level of interest in non-orthodox medicine amongst GPs, with almost half of the general practices in England providing access to CAM in 2001, which can include practitioners actually providing a service such as acupuncture, having CAM practitioners in their clinics or making National Health Service referrals to CAM providers (Sharp et al. 2018). Research in other countries has shown that many orthodox practitioners have an interest in alternative or complementary medicine, such as in the Netherlands (Fisher and Ward 1994), Canada (Verhoef and Sutherland 1998), New Zealand (Poynton et al. 2006), Australia (Wardle et al. 2018), Israel and the United States (Adams 2004) and refer patients on to complementary therapists or practices, and this appears to be becoming more common (Poynton et al. 2006; Sointu 2012). In some areas, nearly half of all nurses use complementary therapies in clinical practice (Shorofi and Arbon 2010).

It would appear from these studies that there is a high level of health professional interest in alternative therapies and a willingness to refer patients on to those who practise an alternative therapy, whether or not they are medically qualified. What we cannot tell from these studies is how much of the doctors' practice is devoted to alternative therapies, although a New Zealand study of doctors trained in acupuncture found that the majority only used the therapy on a small number of patients (Gibb 1988) and a British study of GPs who practised non-orthodox medicine estimated that these therapies were used on no more than five percent of their total number of patients (Sharma 1992). Similarly, although there may be a willingness to refer patients on to those who practise an alternative therapy, the actual incidence of this occurring is probably very low. Chapter 5 provides further detail on the use of CAM practices by orthodox practitioners with the example of medical acupuncturists.

Concluding comments

This chapter has provided an overview of the establishment of a state-recognised medical profession. The idea of orthodoxy, to which alternatives can be contrasted, only came clearly into form when the state conferred power onto a particular body of practitioners who could then determine what was included within state-legitimised therapeutic practices. The exclusion of alternative occupational groupings does not mean that the alternative practices that they use do not find their way into the medical consultation. However, the state establishing a form of statist medicine severely restricts the possibilities of therapeutic pluralism.

Favourable legislation for the medical profession has not been an outcome of proof of effectiveness. This is particularly obvious given that the medical profession triumphed over its rivals in the late nineteenth century when orthodox medicine would be considered by current views as being therapeutically ineffective.

Orthodoxy and effectiveness should not be equated in any simple, linear fashion. Once the medical profession is established as an entity with exclusive boundaries and exclusionary powers, it in effect establishes what is now alternative, irregular and unorthodox. As statist medicine has developed in the West, it has transformed from regular or established medicine to biomedicine. The dominance of understandings of science and technologies that can measure or read the body is central in this development of biomedicine. Therapeutic practices not inside the medical fold are now marginalised because they lack access to the credibility of science. This gets further embedded with the development of evidence-based medicine and the dominance of a specific methodology to determine the effectiveness of treatments, the randomised-controlled trial, one of the practices of disciplining therapeutics that is explored in the following chapter.

References

Abbott, A. (1988) *The system of professions: An essay on the division of expert labor*, Chicago: University of Chicago Press.

Adams, J. (2004) *Demarcating the medical/non-medical border: Occupational boundary-work within GPs' accounts of their integrative practice*, Abingdon, UK: Routledge.

Almeida, J. (2012) The differential incorporation of CAM into the medical establishment: The case of acupuncture and homeopathy in Portugal, *Health Sociology Review*, 765–792.

Beaven, D. (1989) Alternative medicine a cruel hoax: Your money and your life?, *New Zealand Medical Journal*, 102, 873, 416–417.

Belgrave, M. (1985) *'Medical men' and 'lady doctors': The making of a New Zealand profession, 1867–1941*, Ph.D. dissertation, Wellington: Victoria University of Wellington.

Berliner, H. (1984) Scientific medicine since Flexner, in J.W. Salmon (ed.), *Alternative medicines: Popular and policy perspectives*, New York: Tavistock Press, pp. 30–56.

Bivins, R. (2007) *Alternative medicine: A history*, Oxford: Oxford University Press.

Bonderup, G. (2001) Danish society and folk healers 1780–1825, in R. Jütte, M. Eklöf and M. Nelson (eds.), *Historical aspects of unconventional medicine: Approaches, concepts and case studies*, Sheffield: European Association for the History of Medicine and Health Publications, pp. 73–85.

Broom, A., Meurk, C., Adams, J. and Sibbritt, D. (2014) My health, my responsibility? Complementary medicine and self (health) care, *Journal of Sociology*, 50, 4, 515–530.

Brosnan, C. (2015) 'Quackery' in the academy? Professional knowledge, autonomy and the debate over complementary medicine degrees, *Sociology*, 49, 6, 1047–1064.

Cano-Orón, L. (2019) A Twitter campaign against pseudoscience: The sceptical discourse on complementary therapies in Spain, *Public Understanding of Science*, 28, 6, 679–695.

Coulter, H. (1973) *Divided legacy: A history of the schism in medical thought volume one: The patterns emerge: Hippocrates to Paracelsus*, Washington, DC: Wehawken.

——— (1984) Homeopathy, in J.W. Salmon (ed.), *Alternative medicines: Popular and policy perspectives*, New York: Tavistock Press, pp. 57–79.

Dew, K. (2003) *Borderland practices: Regulating alternative therapies in New Zealand*, Dunedin: University of Otago Press.

Dew, K. and Armstrong, L. (n.d.) Can the subaltern heal? Medical marijuana in Aotearoa New Zealand, *Journal of Sociology*, 10.1177/1440783320925144.

Dinges, M. (2001) The contribution of the comparative approach to the history of homeopathy, in R. Jütte, M. Eklöf and M. Nelson (eds.), *Historical aspects of unconventional medicine: Approaches, concepts and case studies*, Sheffield: European Association for the History of Medicine and Health Publications, pp. 51–72.

Duffy, J. (1979) *The healers: A history of American medicine*, Urbana: University of Illinois Press.

Eklöf, M. (2001) Doctor or quack: Legal and lexical definitions in twentieth-century Sweden, in R. Jütte, M. Eklöf and M. Nelson (eds.), *Historical aspects of unconventional medicine: Approaches, concepts and case studies*, Sheffield: European Association for the History of Medicine and Health Publications, pp. 103–117.

Ernst, E. and Smith, K. (2018) *More harm than good? The moral maze of complementary and alternative medicine*, Cham: Springer.

Fisher, P. and Ward, A. (1994) Complementary medicine in Europe, *British Medical Journal*, 309, 107–111.

Foucault, M. (2003) *The birth of the clinic: An archaeology of medical perception*, London and New York: Routledge.

Gevitz, N. (1988) Osteopathic medicine: From deviance to difference, in N. Gevitz (ed.), *Other healers: Unorthodox medicine in America*, Baltimore, MD: John Hopkins University Press, pp. 124–156.

Gibb, G. (1988, April) The development of medical acupuncture in New Zealand, *New Zealand Journal of Acupuncture*, 19–20.

Kaufman, M. (1971) *Homeopathy in America: The rise and fall of a medical heresy*, Baltimore, MD: John Hopkins University Press.

Kelleher, D. (1994) Understanding medical dominance in the modern world, in J. Gabe, D. Kelleher and G. Williams (eds.), *Challenging medicine*, London and New York: Routledge, pp. xi–xxix.

Kelm, M.-E. (2010) Past into present: History and the making of knowledge about HIV/AIDS and Aboriginal people, in D. Herring and A. Swedlund (eds.), *Plagues and epidemics: Infected spaces past and present*, Oxford: Berg, pp. 193–212.

Kenney, C.M. (2011) Midwives, women and families: A Māori gaze, *AlterNative: An International Journal of Indigenous Peoples*, 7, 2, 123–137.

Kneipp, S. (1893[1979]) *My water cure: The famous system of healing developed and practised in the nineteenth century by Pfarrer Kneipp at his parish at Worishofen in Bavaria*, Wellingborough: Thorsons.

Lange, R. (1999) *May the people live: A history of Māori health development 1900–1920*, Auckland: Auckland University Press.

Larkin, G. (1983) *Occupational monopoly and modern medicine*, London: Tavistock Press.

Ling, S. (2001) Physicians, quacks and the field of medicine: A case study of quackery in nineteenth-century Sweden, in R. Jütte, M. Eklöf and M. Nelson (eds.), *Historical aspects of unconventional medicine: Approaches, concepts and case studies*, Sheffield: European Association for the History of Medicine and Health Publications, pp. 87–102.

Nicholls, P. (1988) *Homoeopathy and the medical profession*, London: Croom Helm.

——— (2001) The social construction and organisation of medical marginality: The case of homeopathy in mid nineteenth century Britain, in R. Jütte, M. Eklöf and M. Nelson (eds.), *Historical aspects of unconventional medicine: Approaches, concepts and case studies*, Sheffield: European Association for the History of Medicine and Health Publications, pp. 163–181.

Nutton, V. (1995a) Medicine in medieval Western Europe, 1000–1500, in L. Conrad (ed.), *The Western medical tradition: 800 AD to AD 1800*, Cambridge: Cambridge University Press, pp. 139–205.

——— (1995b) Roman medicine, 250 BC to AD 200, in L. Conrad (ed.), *The Western medical tradition: 800 BC to AD 1800*. Cambridge: Cambridge University Press, pp. 39–70.

Pétursdóttir, S.S. (2001) Homeopathy in Iceland, in R. Jütte, M. Eklöf and M. Nelson (eds.), *Historical aspects of unconventional medicine: Approaches, concepts, case studies*, Sheffield: European Association for the History of Medicine and Health Publications, pp. 183–192.

Pokladnikova, J. and Telec, I. (2020) Provision of complementary and alternative medicine: Compliance with the health professional requirements, *Health Policy*, 124, 3, 311–316.

Poynton, L., Dowell, A., Dew, K. and Egan, T. (2006) General practitioners' attitudes toward (and use of) complementary and alternative medicine: A New Zealand nationwide survey, *New Zealand Medical Journal*, 119, 1247.

Rosenberg, C.E. (1987) *The care of strangers: The rise of the America's hospital system*, New York: Basic Books.

——— (1992) *Explaining epidemics and other studies in the history of medicine*, Cambridge: Cambridge University Press.

Rothstein, W. (1988) The botanical movements and orthodox Medicine, in N. Gevitz (ed.), *Other healers: Unorthodox medicine in America*, Baltimore, MD: John Hopkins University Press, pp. 29–51.

Sharma, S. (1992) *Complementary medicine today: Practitioners and patients*, London: Routledge.

Sharp, D., Lorenc, A., Little, P., Mercer, S.W., Hollinghurst, S., Feder, G. and MacPherson, H. (2018) Complementary medicine and the NHS: Experiences of integration with UK primary care, *European Journal of Integrative Medicine*, 24, 8–16.

Shorofi, S.A. and Arbon, P. (2010) Nurses' knowledge, attitude and professional use of complementary and alternative medicine (CAM): A survey of five metropolitan hospitals in Adelaide, *Complementary Therapies in Clinical Practice*, 16, 4, 229–234.

Sigsworth, E.M. (1972) Gateways to death? Medicine, hospitals and mortality, 1700–1850, in P. Mathias (ed.), *Science and society 1600–1900*, Cambridge: Cambridge University Press, pp. 97–110.

Sointu, E. (2012) *Theorizing complementary and alternative medicines: Wellbeing, self, gender, class*, Basingstoke: Palgrave.

Starr, P. (1982) *The social transformation of American medicine*, New York: Basic Books.

Stolberg, M. (2001) Alternative medicine, irregular healers and the medical market in nineteenth-century Bavaria, in R. Jütte, M. Eklöf and M. Nelson (eds.), *Historical aspects of unconventional medicine: Approaches, concepts and case studies*, Sheffield: European Association for the History of Medicine and Health Publications, pp. 139–162.

Verhoef, M.J. and Sutherland, L.R. (1998) Alternative medicine and general practitioners: Opinions and behaviour, *Complementary Therapies in Medicine*, 6, 2, 108–109.

Waddington, I. (1977) General practitioners and consultants in early nineteenth-century England: The sociology of an intra-professional conflict, in J. Woodward and D. Richards (eds.), *Health care in popular medicine in nineteenth century England*, London: Croom Helm, pp. 164–188.

Wardle, J.L., Sibbritt, D.W. and Adams, J. (2018) Primary care practitioner perceptions and attitudes of complementary medicine: A content analysis of free-text responses from a survey of non-metropolitan Australian general practitioners, *Primary Health Care Research & Development*, 19, 3, 246–255.

Wear, A. (1995) Medicine in early modern Europe, 1500–1700, in L.I. Conrad (ed.), *The Western medical tradition: 800 BC to AD 1800*, Cambridge: Cambridge University Press, pp. 215–361.

Willis, E. (1983) *Medical dominance: The division of labour in Australian healthcare*, Sydney: George Allen & Unwin.

3

DISCIPLINING AND INTEGRATING PRACTICES

There are many factors that impact upon the availability of therapeutic modalities, whether CAM or orthodox, and the use of particular therapeutic interventions (e.g., using medication when a diagnosis of diabetes is made or using changes in diet and exercise). In Chapter 2, the importance of state recognition and the standardisation of education are discussed. But with that state benefit comes the possibility of increasing forms of state control over therapeutic practices, which can impact on the autonomy of the medical profession, the major beneficiaries of state largesse. Regulation of the medical profession, where limitations are placed on who can call themselves doctors and what doctors can do, is a double-edged sword. Regulation can provide legitimacy, but it can limit therapeutic freedom and autonomy. If the medical profession integrates with the state to gain a monopoly over medical practice, then one consequence is that the autonomous power of the medical profession is limited. That is, the state has the potential to put pressure on the profession, for example, putting in place health commissioners that can rule on patient complaints about medical professionals. The forms that this pressure takes can then have consequences for those therapeutic practitioners who are not so embedded in the state and who are not part of the medical profession, such as CAM practitioners. As such, the impact of statist medicine can shape and potentially limit therapeutic possibilities beyond the direct reach of the state.

Since the late 1970s, there has been a worldwide phenomenon of attempts by the state to control an ever-increasing demand for healthcare resources. This followed a period of expansion of the health sector and an optimistic attitude that health services would vastly improve the health of the population. By the 1970s, it became apparent that medicine could absorb resources indefinitely, and yet the returns were diminishing and major health problems remained (Marmor et al. 1994).

These concerns over expenditure facilitated the rise of health economics (Berg 1997). Different forms of priority setting in the health sector have followed, where efforts can direct resources to therapeutic products and interventions that are regarded as being of the most benefit. Those activities that give the most life years at high quality for the least cost will be prioritised (Tenbensel 2000). Efforts to determine what interventions provide the most benefit have supported the development and empowerment of what is known as the evidence-based medicine movement. The dominance of evidence-based medicine means that those interventions that most readily accommodate a hierarchy of evidence can become the focus of prioritisation. These developments further marginalise CAM. A central and crucial aspect of these processes of marginalisation of CAM and the prioritisation of therapeutic interventions is the randomised controlled trial (RCT).

Therapeutic credibility and RCTs

A powerful mechanism, in practice and used rhetorically, enabling the continued subordination of alternative practices to a medical orthodoxy is the status given to the double-blind placebo-controlled trial, which I will refer to as the RCT. In terms of contemporary standards, any substances used by medical practitioners in the nineteenth century were not standardised. Therefore, practitioners could only estimate the potency of the substances they were giving. It was not until the twentieth century that the medical research 'style of reasoning' (Hacking 1990) that underpinned the RCT developed.

In 1910, the idea of the 'biological assay' was suggested. The biological assay is a test performed to measure the biological activity of a drug or remedy, and the idea of the assay was proposed by American authors writing in the *American Journal of Pharmacy*. Biological activity relates to the effect and potency of a remedy. In 1910, it was suggested that the biological potency of digitalis (from the leaves of the foxglove) could be assessed by a 'cat unit' (Porter 1995). That is, pharmacists making up the potion could test the potency of the leaves by finding out how many leaves it took to kill a cat (Porter 1995). This effort to find the strength of medicinal preparations had limitations as different cats varied in their tolerance for drugs. But the concept of the biological assay paved the way for attempts to standardise medicines, and it was not until medicines themselves were standardised that one could put any faith in tests of therapeutic effectiveness.

Without standardising the drug, you could not tell whether the effect of giving the drug (whether negative or positive) was a result of the regimen of treatment per se or of the potency of the dose you gave. If the dose varied at each treatment, there might sometimes be no effect, sometimes the effect desired and sometimes adverse effects depending on whether the potency was weak, about right or too strong. The focus here is on the use of drugs and an assumption that different people will react in the same or very similar ways to the same, standardised drug. Once drugs are standardised, the possibility of comparing one group of people who receive the drug with another group who do not receive it becomes meaningful. However, in the nineteenth century, as medicine was increasingly given state patronage, the idea that statistical methods should be employed to determine the efficacy of a treatment was resisted by physicians (Porter 1995). To accept the notion of a controlled trial would be to subordinate clinical judgements and medical ideas to the dominance of numbers. Claude Bernard, a famous nineteenth-century French advocate of experimental research, abhorred statistical inquiries: 'He wanted to examine the specific lesions and injuries to organs, not the average of many organs' (Hacking 1990: 71). Attempts in the early twentieth century to use statistical tests to assess the outcomes of treatments undermined the central place of the individual patient, the focus of medical attention, and so was rejected (Hacking 1990: 85). It was not until the 1940s that statistical tests gained a firm foothold in medical research.

The idea of comparing groups to look for statistically significant differences was a style of reasoning that was foreign and alien to nineteenth-century medical men. A great many more concepts needed to be accepted before clinical trials could become the norm. One important concept was the notion of 'normal' that could be compared with the deviant (Hacking 1990). Without a notion of a normal distribution of the population, it was not possible to establish whether the responses one got from a therapeutic intervention were due to chance (therefore not outside the normal distribution) or due to some real effect (therefore 'deviating' in a positive way from a normal distribution). The notion of 'normal' that we use today did not take a hold on medical and social thought until the late nineteenth century.

With the standardising of drugs and the acceptance of the concept of a normal distribution, the methodology of the RCT could be developed. In the RCT, one group of people receives the treatment and another group does not. For all people in the trial to have a similar experience and a similar set of expectations, neither group should know whether they are receiving the treatment or not. So, the non-treatment group is given a placebo, or an inert or inactive pill. The placebo effect is a well-known phenomenon, in which people gain a positive therapeutic outcome even though no active treatment has been given. The placebo effect is very real and, depending on the condition being treated and a host of other variables can have a forty percent success rate. This power that we have in ourselves to heal if we believe in the therapeutic process must be controlled for in determining the effectiveness of a particular substance. For it to have value, the trialled treatment has to perform better than placebo.

The RCT now sits at the top of the hierarchy of evidence-based medicine, and as such is used by champions of orthodox medicine to attack the credibility of any therapeutic system that has not successfully passed the RCT test. However, RCTs were not designed to test the efficacy of all therapeutic practices. They were designed to test the efficacy of pharmaceuticals. The first RCT occurred in 1946 to evaluate the use of streptomycin in the treatment of pulmonary tuberculosis (Porter 2006). The thalidomide tragedy of the 1950s and

1960s provided a strong impetus for the uptake of RCTs before drugs came onto the market. In this tragedy, tens of thousands of babies throughout the world were born with serious birth defects after their mothers took the pharmaceutical during pregnancy (Light 2010). This mechanism for assessing dangerous drugs has become the standard that all therapeutic interventions are expected to pass. However, many therapeutic approaches, orthodox and alternative, cannot readily meet the requirements of RCTs. In the double-blind trial, the person performing the therapeutic act should not know whether they are giving the patient the real treatment or a placebo, because if they do know then that might influence, whether consciously or not, how the patient responds to the treatment. For many practitioners, such as psychotherapists, body therapists and acupuncturists, what they do requires a level of skill and expertise, so they will know if they are providing a real treatment or not. By contrast, giving someone a pill requires no skill or expertise (although of course making a diagnosis requires expertise).

Even for therapeutic approaches that use pills, the processes by which a particular pill is decided upon may make the approach difficult to assess using RCTs. Homeopaths can use remedies in pill form; however, homeopathy's philosophy of diagnosing and prescribing is not the same as it is with orthodox practitioners. Orthodox medical practitioners diagnose a condition, say migraine, and prescribe a medication that would be the same for all those who have the same condition. Therefore, a trial can be conducted on all migraine patients because they would all get the same medication. Homeopaths diagnose and prescribe on the basis of finding a single remedy that is right for that person, not the condition. Two people with migraine might then get different remedies. To test the homeopathic remedies by RCT does not then make sense. Another difficulty for CAM therapeutic practices is that conducting RCTs is a very expensive process and requires the backing of corporations who will look forward to large returns on their investment, which is based on being able to patent pharmaceuticals. Rewards for homeopathic remedies would not return that investment.

In many countries, the state has actively supported the unlevel therapeutic testing playing field. For example, in 2000, a House of Lords report in the United Kingdom concluded that CAM needed to build up its evidence base in the same way as biomedicine – with a focus on RCTs (Jackson and Scambler 2007), in effect ignoring the inappropriate match between a therapy and a research design.

It is clear then that one important way to marginalise alternative therapies is to require them to conform to a research methodology, or a test of efficacy, that was not designed for these alternative therapies, but was designed for dangerously potent pharmaceuticals. The emphasis placed on RCTs as a marker of therapeutic credibility is an extremely powerful means of limiting therapeutic pluralism. Other developments in the regulation of professions entwines with this evidence-based medicine rhetoric to further disadvantage CAM in clinical and educational settings, as well as politically.

Regulation

Priority setting in government spending can directly and indirectly impact upon accessibility of CAM to the citizenry, and priority-setting and guidelines related to state spending have been influenced by the evidence-based medicine movement.

The rise of evidence-based medicine is a consequence of a number of goals. One is to provide credibility to the medical profession by claiming that interventions are backed up by the best science. Another is that evidence can lead to guidelines or recommendations being developed, so that variation in clinical practice can be reduced. Evidence can also feed into calculations about what services are cost-effective and so whether they should be provided in a public system or not. Evidence-based medicine developed in an effort to orient medicine towards what was perceived as the existing science and knowledge base. It became increasingly important in the 1990s, although a milestone text was Archie Cochrane's 1972 text *Effectiveness and Efficacy* (Cochrane 1972). At the top of the evidence-based medicine hierarchy of evidence for interventions is the RCT while the bottom level is where guidelines are based on the consensus of experts. Although advocates of evidence-based medicine argue that decisions should be based on the most appropriate evidence, therefore potentially extending beyond RCTs in the context of interventions, RCTs still dominate systematic reviews aimed at influencing treatment decision-making (Green 2000).

Health economists have strongly criticised the clinical autonomy of medical practitioners as it undermines the efficient allocation of health resources (Maynard 1995). In order to combat this wasteful use of resources, health economists have developed systems to quantify health outcomes, so that costs can be effectively related to them (Ashmore et al. 1989; Seedhouse 1995). A central component of this strategy is to include the use of RCTs to determine effectiveness and, failing that, the use of 'experts' to develop a consensus. The consensus then forms the basis of quality assurance procedures with which practitioners are expected to conform. Concern over the variability of practice promotes attempts to constrain the medical profession and to standardise medical practices. Reducing practitioner variability and creating homogeneity across the professions advance greater levels of professional control (Frenk and Durán-Arenas 1993), and this homogeneity is in conflict with both the individual practitioner's clinical freedom and reduces the therapeutic possibilities available to patients.

Linking evidence-based medicine to forms of professional accountability then restricts the art of medicine and the autonomy of the practitioner. Scholars have drawn on Max Weber's concepts in arguing that evidence-based practice undermines traditional clinical expertise as clinicians are increasingly required to point to an external evidentiary authority in order to provide justification for their decisions, as opposed to relying on their own experience (Lipman 2000). Managers and bureaucracies oversee and control the implementation of evidence-based practice, further undermining the clinical autonomy of practitioners (Checkland et al. 2008; Lipman 2000).

Codes of conduct and professional standards, including guidelines, protocols and practice policies, are some of the bureaucratic means of gaining conformity to evidence-based findings. These bureaucratic means are 'instructions telling medical personnel to do a certain thing in a certain situation' (Berg 1997: 2). Medical practice can then be more standardised and defined as the logical and sequential application of science.

The requirement to 'rein in' the individual practitioner is in part a response to burgeoning healthcare costs burdening the state. As the state looks to limit this burden, the medical profession responds by putting its own house in order. State authorities may attempt to control the content of medical practice in a number of ways, including the laying down of explicit guidelines for medical practice (Coburn et al. 1997). Quality improvement schemes applied to the delivery of healthcare services have been developed to improve accountability and further standardise therapeutic practices. Quality assurance programmes set standards and assess medical professionals against those standards. If compliance to the standards is not achieved, then corrective action can be taken to discipline the practitioner (Jost 1992: 70). Quality assurance programmes can include peer reviews of practitioners by colleagues or by external agents, individual practitioner medical audits, continuing medical education and other activities.

Prior to the 1980s, there were no explicit references made to quality assurance in health care, though systems for specifying, checking and maintaining quality had been developing since the 1960s in Britain and the United States, due to the increasing costs of health services (Ellis and Whittington 1993). Quality assurance developments in England were the result of, on the one hand, governmental concerns with efficiency, consumer service, business-like management and accountability in the National Health Service, and on the other the drive by Royal Colleges and others to improve the practice of medicine (Jost 1992). The method of medical audit comes from the United States, where insurance companies imposed audits upon doctors in order to limit the cost of medical care (Seale 1993).

It is not until the 1980s that we start to see efforts being made to try to ensure that doctors remain competent to practice after receiving their medical license (Chamberlain 2013). Atrocity stories about medical practice have facilitated this process, such as the Shipman case in the United Kingdom. Dr Shipman was a GP in the Greater Manchester area. It was found that Shipman had murdered at least 215 elderly patients over a period of about 25 years (Chamberlain 2013). The case is an extreme one, but it supported calls for the introduction of systems of quality assurance and accountability, such as the revalidation of practitioners to test their clinical competence on a regular basis. As a result of the range of quality assurance programmes that have been introduced, like revalidation, the professional autonomy of individual practitioners has been limited.

The development of quality assurance in medical practice does not undermine the dominance of the medical profession in relation to other professions. Through controlling the work of individual medical practitioners, quality assurance preserves the power for the medical profession as a whole (Coburn et al. 1997). In addition, accountability and assurance mechanisms reinforce the paradigm of biomedicine in the delivery of health services. It does this by limiting what individual practitioners can do and imposing similar quality assurance mechanisms on other therapeutic modalities desiring to gain state resources. One resource that many CAM professional organisations seek is state regulation. The Osteopaths Act of 1993 in the United Kingdom noted in the previous chapter is an example as obtaining this resource of state regulation enabled state-recognised osteopathic organisations to protect the title osteopath. That is, to determine whether someone would be able to call themselves an osteopath. Such regulation brings the CAM groupings into the orbit of statist medicine and its auditing and standardising culture.

These developments may take a toll on those individual practitioners who attempt to develop different paths to the provision of health care. Whether it is management or a medical elite that gains increasing influence over the content of clinical practice, the effect is likely to be similar. Practitioners who do something different, such as using acupuncture or, even more challengingly, homeopathy, have the prospect of the efficiency and effectiveness of their practices being assessed by peers or managers. One outcome is that this can detract from consumer choice and limit the availability of alternative forms of treatment that are not susceptible to standardised trials and do not conform to current orthodox beliefs about disease.

The language of health economics is not so easy to employ by those outside of the medical profession practising alternative therapies. Quantifying the impact of CAM treatments is not a simple matter as the use of RCTs rarely fits the paradigm within which they operate. Without being able to reach this gold standard of proving therapeutic efficacy, gaining access to political resources is much more difficult.

What we see in these developments with the medical profession is increasing control over what practitioners can do and the enshrining of 'objective' criteria in processes that dictate what practitioners can do. These developments have spilled out to impact on CAM health practitioners. For example, in the New Zealand context, a Health Practitioners Competence Assurance Act was legislated in 2003. This Act is modelled on a prior Medical Practitioners Act and includes competence and re-certification programmes that practitioners are required to undertake under the oversight of their own associations, and some CAM groupings including chiropractors and osteopaths are contained in the Act. As CAM practitioners attempt to access the resources of the state, they are drawn into mechanisms of state control. A quite different mechanism of controlling CAM can be seen in the attempts to integrate CAM with mainstream medicine.

Integrating practices in education

Significant efforts to institutionalise the integration of CAM and biomedical practices started to take shape in the 1970s. In 1978, the American Holistic

Medical Association was established by biomedical practitioners and American osteopaths, and in 1995, the American Holistic Nurses Association was established, and nursing schools started to offer courses in alternative therapies (Baer and Coulter 2008). Andrew Weil, who is credited with coining the term integrative medicine, established a programme in integrative medicine at the University of Arizona in 1994, aimed at family practitioners and internists interested in incorporating alternative medicine into their conventional practices (Baer and Coulter 2008). There was a rapid rise in the teaching of CAM or integrative medicine courses in the United States going from twenty-six percent of medical schools offering required courses in 2001 to ninety-one percent in 2009 (Possamai-Inesedy and Cochrane 2013). In 2007, over one-third of US hospitals offered at least one integrative therapy service (Possamai-Inesedy and Cochrane 2013).

CAM has then been integrated to some extent, or in some instances, into Western educational systems. In one study of the research and teaching of CAM at university level, Caragh Brosnan (2016) identified different epistemic cultures at play in relation to TCM and osteopathy taught in universities. Epistemic cultures, a term taken from Karin Knorr-Cetina, refer to different branches of science that have different machineries of knowing, and therefore different values and practices. In Chinese medicine courses, it was found that lecturers were engaged in biomedically shaped evidence-based processes, particularly the RCT but also laboratory-based research, to build up an evidence base that would be convincing to the public, to sceptics and to funders. As such, these academics were conforming to the disciplinary and regulatory practices of statist medicine, and so engaged in the reshaping of TCM to align with these disciplinary practices.

Brosnan contrasts this with the desire in osteopathic courses for more diverse forms of assessment, such as qualitative assessment that included patients' perceptions and experiences. This latter has also been called for by social science researchers who suggest that the complexity of CAM therapeutics means more diverse assessment methods are required if we are to gain a better understanding of CAM efficacy (Possamai-Inesedy and Cochrane 2013). To accept more diverse forms of assessment would dethrone the RCT, and in doing so open up a credible field of therapeutics beyond the biomedical reliance on pharmaceuticals.

Back in the universities' Chinese medicine classrooms, theories of Chinese medicine were used in teaching, including the use of such concepts as qi and the functional anatomy used in TCM, without reference to Western medicine. In effect, students were taught to compartmentalise these different understandings. The epistemic culture of research was in fact quite different from the epistemic culture of teaching, where the former was aimed at the public and the latter was for the practitioners to be (Brosnan 2016). These mechanisms of compartmentalisation also occur in non-Western countries, where different therapeutic systems challenge the dominance of biomedicine, such as in China (see Scheid 2002; discussed in Chapter 5) and in India (see Langford 2002; discussed in Chapter 6).

This trend towards the incorporation of CAM practices into institutional fora has met with a strong backlash in some jurisdictions. In December 2011, the Friends of Science and Medicine was established in Australia by thirty-four Australian doctors and scientists in response to their concerns about the acceptance and prevalence of CAM in Australia (Lewis 2019). In 2012, the Friends of Science and Medicine lobbied for the abolition of CAM courses from Australian universities (Possamai-Inesedy and Cochrane 2013), with its first media release objecting to the introduction of a Bachelor of Science (Chiropractic) at Central Queensland University. The Friends of Science and Medicine continued to lobby to remove the teaching of CAM from universities. Their campaign included writing to the vice chancellors of Australian universities with questions about their teaching of CAM and whether they ensured their health-related courses were evidence-based (Brosnan 2015). Press releases stating that CAM teaching had no place in universities gained media coverage and initiated responses from vice chancellors and others defending their curricula. The Friends of Science and Medicine campaigned on two major planks: (1) CAM degrees give credibility to pseudoscience with bioscience being the only means to academic legitimacy in the health sciences and (2) the reputation of Australian universities would be undermined if they continued to teach CAM (Brosnan 2015). Brosnan argues that in this we see that the Friends of Science and Medicine fear that the dominant values in university therapeutic training that they are privileged by are being threatened by those in subordinate positions (Brosnan 2015). If CAM was successful, then the notion of one universal form of knowledge would be undermined and alternative ways of knowing would be legitimised.

However, the public defence to these attacks from the universities was not to promote CAM practices as an alternative, perhaps holistic, paradigm, but to claim that CAM degrees were strongly based in bioscience, and because of this scientific training, the CAM practitioners who would hold their degrees would be able to practice safely, in contrast to those fringe practitioners without university degrees (Brosnan 2015). CAM was then positioned in these defences as being aligned with biomedicine and statist medicine, based on the values of biomedicine, and so posing no threat to the dominant paradigm.

The impact of campaigns like the Friends of Science and Medicine is difficult to assess. The Friends of Science and Medicine claimed success when one university closed a degree course in chiropractic, but the university itself situated this closure as a result of a desire to focus on more research-intensive areas (Brosnan 2015). This points to another means by which CAM may be increasingly marginalised in the education system, with the importance placed on STEM subjects, science, technology, engineering and medicine, in terms of state funding, and universities having their ranking influenced by research outputs, possibly side-lining CAM approaches that are, as yet, not likely to be competitive in relation to other subjects with higher levels of research activity. For example, it is far less likely that CAM research will be successful in competitive funding models than biomedical or public health research if, for no other reason, than the assessors of such research applications are primarily drawn from biomedical and public health fields and are not CAM academics.

Another way of measuring the impact of the Friends of Science and Medicine is to assess the voice it gained in the Australian media. The Friends of Science and Medicine, even though a relatively small group (with 400 members by 2018), was able to get its message across in very robust fashion. Where the Friends of Science and Medicine was mentioned in the media, this was overwhelmingly in articles that had negative headlines and a negative tone about CAM, in particular framing CAM as a lucrative and unethical industry and as an illegitimate pseudoscience (Lewis 2019). The Friends of Science and Medicine spokespeople were prominent in these articles with very little representation from other potentially relevant experts such as CAM researchers. These findings suggest that journalists, in Australia at least, readily adopt the assumptions and views of privileged groups defending a particular medical and scientific orthodoxy (Lewis 2019). It also signals the readiness of the media to homogenise the incredible diversity of CAM practices.

In Spain, there have been recent formations of sceptics groups with the explicit aim of countering the promotion of CAM (Cano-Orón 2019). Their activities are wide-ranging, including protesting at presentations on CAM topics and trying to prevent such presentations from going ahead, and setting up search engines, so that people can identify pharmacies that do not sell homeopathic products (Cano-Orón 2019). As with the Friends of Science and Medicine influence on Australian journalists, these groups have had a major impact on Spanish journalists, but also on politicians wary of being the target of social media campaigns from such groups if they did not discourage CAM. Spanish political parties have made proposals that would make health professionals report what are deemed pseudoscientific practices, and all the main political parties have distanced themselves from CAM (Cano-Orón 2019).

These examples clearly indicate a powerful form of disciplinary practice, where anti-CAM lobby groups have been able to exert powerful influences over the media and politicians, and foster an environment that is hostile to CAM, potentially reducing state support, research activities and educational opportunities for CAM disciplines.

Clinical integration

Integrative medicine references situations where conventional and alternative medical practices may be available through the one clinical practice or even the one clinical practitioner. However, integrative medicine tends to be on the terms of conventional medicine where, for example, CAM may be added into hospital-based programmes, or CAM can be claimed by conventional medicine if it is shown to pass the rigours of the conventional evidence-based medicine hierarchy (Coulter 2004). Some medical practitioners claim that CAM practices can be reconfigured in orthodox medical terms and so be legitimately used in medical practice. The needling used in acupuncture is thought to act on entities like qi and meridians according to TCM, but Western medical acupuncturists can claim that needling acts in a conventional physiological way by, for example, releasing endorphins (Dew 2000). This Western explanation became available from the late twentieth century with the discovery of endorphins.

In the 1990s, a number of integrative medical clinics were established in the United States, although support for CAM activities in these clinics was compromised because of the labour-intensive approaches of CAM compared to biomedical care (Baer and Coulter 2008), an issue further commented on in Chapter 7. In 1991, the first alternative health clinic was opened in a government hospital in Israel (Mizrachi et al. 2005). Ten years later in a study of acupuncturists operating inside a government hospital in Tel Aviv, it was found that they were in a very marginal position, offering their services voluntarily and being assigned under biomedical authority to treat only particular conditions. Alternative practitioners rendered their services free of charge as they saw themselves as pioneering and having an opportunity to gain legitimacy in the biomedical setting (Mizrachi et al. 2005). The subordination of alternative approaches to biomedicine, even where integration is claimed, is evident in many settings.

In North America, Integrated Medicine centres have arisen that are condition specific, such as for cancer or chronic pain (Hollenberg and Muzzin 2010). In a Canadian study, Daniel Hollenberg and Linda Muzzin show how CAM practices can be marginalised in relation to biomedical practices in these settings. At a multidisciplinary pain management centre in a Canadian hospital, acupuncturists trained in TCM worked alongside biomedical practitioners. In an interview, a biomedical practitioner at the site equated acupuncture with chicken soup – in that it could 'do a lot of good, it can't do any harm' (Hollenberg and Muzzin 2010: 43). This analogy suggests something that is comforting, maybe nourishing, rather than having the kudos of being clinically effective. Many things could act like chicken soup. In addition, at this site, none of the biomedical practitioners understood the TCM diagnosis given to the patients and they would use the diagnosis coming from the biomedical paradigm. The effects of acupuncture would be described in biomedical terms, such as the release of pain-relieving endorphins, rather than in TCM terms, and would only be considered as useful for specific conditions such as muscle pain. Although acupuncture was allowed the use of Chinese herbs and moxibustion was not (there is further discussion of these practices in Chapter 5).

Alongside the subordination of CAM practices in 'integrated settings', there has been an increasing interest in providing CAM services alongside biomedical ones. In 2001, around fifty percent of general practices in England provided access to CAM services, an increase from thirty-eight percent in 1995 (Sharp et al. 2018). The provision could take different shapes. GPs or nurses could provide the service directly, with the most common therapy used being acupuncture. CAM practitioners could be based in the general practice, with the most common ones being manipulative therapists. Or referrals could be made on to

CAM providers that would be covered by the National Health Service. Around twenty percent of UK physicians provided CAM in their practice in any one week.

In Australia, claims have been made that medical doctors are increasingly prescribing herbal products, but that this is a case of mainstreaming of an alternative approach by co-option (Singer and Fisher 2007). That is, prescribing is based on a biomedical approach to reduce symptoms as opposed to traditional herbalist approaches to restore balance and appeal to the vital forces of the body. Another indicator of co-option is name changes that have occurred in the training of herbalists, where the more scientifically sounding term of phytotherapy is used (Singer and Fisher 2007).

In China, in the 1980s, Integrated Chinese and Western medicine was officially supported, along with standalone Chinese Medicine and Western medicine (see Chapter 5). The way this is used varies. It can mean the uptake of Western medicine practices by Chinese medicine physicians or the uptake of Chinese medicine practices by Western medicine physicians. It can refer to an ideal of creating a new medicine that develops out of the integration of Chinese and Western medicine, and it can mean the institutions and hospitals that train physicians in integrated medicine and publish research on it (Scheid 2002). Volker Scheid argues that in practice education efforts directed at integrated medicine in China are undertaken by Chinese medicine institutions and not biomedical ones. This suggests the dominance of biomedicine in China, where Chinese medicine can extend out into efforts to integrate Western biomedicine, but this is not so readily reciprocated.

However, practitioners of an integrated medicine in China can position their approach as superior because to rely on Western medicine alone is to rely on an approach that has a good grasp on isolated areas but not complex processes and to rely on Chinese medicine is to ignore the advances made in scientific medicine (Scheid 2002). An integrated physician observed by Scheid would combine biomedicine and Chinese medicine in treating the one patient. Sometimes the biomedical drug was used to have a quick impact then Chinese herbs used to consolidate the treatment, and sometimes biomedicine would be used to treat a particular 'isolated' condition like hypertension, and Chinese medicine used to treat the cause as identified through Chinese medical diagnosis, such as kidney yin depletion (Scheid 2002). Chinese medical practitioners in China can combine Western ideas about drug effects into herbal formulations that are based on the assumptions of Chinese medicine. Western anatomical and physiological understandings of disease causation can be conceptually linked to the functional body (referring to such aspects as functional, but non-anatomical, substances and organs in the body) of Chinese medicine. The use of biomedical understandings, tests and prescriptions can be used in ways to confirm the understandings in ancient Chinese medical texts and also to open up new approaches to treatment (Scheid 2002). There is then, for many Chinese medical practices, a dynamic process of interaction and transformation, and not the static application of formulas based on the Chinese medical archives. Scheid (2002) argues that there is no single medical system in which these Chinese medicine physicians operate, rather physicians enact therapeutic pluralist practices.

In the clinical setting, we see a great variety of 'integrating' practices. They can range from practitioners that reshape alternative practices into the terms of biomedicine through to biomedical technologies used to enhance alternative practices. But people who use these services do so deploying their own forms of integration.

People who seek out therapeutic intervention for conditions they identify as needing some external help have their own ways of integrating orthodox and alternative medicines (see Chapter 7 on users). Research on household use of medications shows how people mix and match different therapies, try out different approaches and take advice from many sources including family, friends, work colleagues, as well as health practitioners both orthodox and unorthodox. Through this process, people may establish regimes that suit their own sense of what is beneficial and that align with their own values and assumptions (Chamberlain et al. 2011; Dew et al. 2014). That is, users of medications take a pragmatic approach, mixing different health approaches particularly in the face of chronic conditions. This mixing and matching also happens in cultures with indigenous healing practices. For example, Tibetans will draw on Tibetan medicine particularly for chronic conditions but also use biomedical approaches (Janes 2002). This is further discussed in Chapter 5 in relation to Chinese medicine and Chapter 6 in relation to therapeutic practices in India.

Understanding the mainstreaming of CAM

Social science perspectives on the incorporation of CAM into biomedicine vary widely. Christopher Fries argues that integrated medicine represents an expansion of medical influences into all domains of human life, based around neo-liberal conceptions of the autonomous individual, but one that is compelled by discourses of wellness (Fries 2008). This is a Foucauldian-influenced orientation suggesting that the rise of CAM and of the concept of integrated medicine are manifestations of new forms of governance.

Others argue that the trends that promote the use of CAM relate more to the operations of capitalism. Historically CAM practitioners have been small business operators with little in the way of state interference. However, by the end of the twentieth century, there was apparent a trend of CAM practitioners becoming employers of larger companies with, for example, naturopaths being employed by supplement and vitamin companies or even pharmaceutical companies in Australia (Collyer 2004). Pharmaceutical companies also distribute CAM products. The expansion of CAM products into supermarkets and pharmacies is one manifestation of these developments in the corporatisation of CAM. Fran Collyer (2004) argues that CAM is now a part of mainstream corporate activity.

David Hess (2004) suggests that since the 1960s there has been a process of medical modernisation in which epistemic changes have occurred in the medical profession. He argues that there has been a shift, to a greater or lesser degree, from the extremes of paternalistic progressivism, which emphasises the purity of science and may actively suppress the challenges and knowledge claims of CAM, and medical devolutionists, a radical extreme of CAM, that rejects mainstream medicine as corrupt and materialistic. Medical modernisation is a process of incorporating aspects of CAM and of (some) funding of CAM research as an outcome of several processes. The most common process is what Hess refers to as a network assemblage, where CAM activists establish networks of patients, funders, practitioners (medical and CAM) and researchers (Hess 2004). An illustrative example of such a process is CAM cancer nutritional therapies. Lobbying from network assemblages promoted funding support for research through the National Center for Complementary and Alternative Medicine of the National Institute of Health in the United States, with other funding coming from the supplements industry and others. As knowledge claims around the role of nutrition in cancer built up and became embedded in consensus statements and review essays, the attempts to undermine such claims by the paternalistic progressives lost ground. From such developments, new entities emerged, like nutraceuticals. The establishment of alternative research networks then led to new research programmes within the medical establishment – the kind of change that Hess (2004) refers to as medical modernisation.

Another mechanism of integration can come from efforts to confront the impact of colonialism in health outcomes and healthcare delivery. In the latter part of the twentieth century, there was, for indigenous peoples of Australasia and North America, a cultural revival or renaissance, which included political lobbying for the recognition of indigenous cultures and languages (Pearson 2001). Land rights movements became more prominent, making claims on dispossessed lands or compensation for that dispossession, and accompanying this with calls for greater autonomy and self-determination, including the delivery of social and health services.

Relationships between the state, biomedicine and indigenous healing systems play out differently in the colonial and settler societies of North America and Australasia than it does in the Indian subcontinent, the latter discussed in Chapter 6. In settler societies, there are some similarities, such as periods of suppression and periods of, at least, partial recognition of indigenous health systems. But the level of state recognition has been much more haphazard, and, to date, there has been no sense of an overarching strategy to promote or research indigenous healing systems in these colonised countries.

In more recent times, measures have been taken by health authorities to empower indigenous groups. During the interwar years, public health interventions in rural areas of Europe and the Americas supported indigenous development (Murard 2008). Since the 1970s, there has been increasing interest in drawing on indigenous health understandings to respond to health problems in the indigenous community, with a particular flourishing of healing and spiritual practices in drug and alcohol treatment programmes in Canada and the United States (Brady 1995). For example, the high rates of alcohol-related illness and death amongst indigenous populations in North America and Australia have led to a restoration of healing practices which are grounded in the view that substance abuse is at least partially an outcome of cultural disruption, or a result of a rejection of the 'culture of the colonizers' (Brady 1995: 1487).

Developments in North America have been taken up by other indigenous peoples, such as indigenous Australians, although the Australian government was far more reticent in embracing such moves than the Canadian government (Brady 1995). Concerns have been raised that the way that the concept of culture that has been used in treatment programmes equates more with the idea of an authentic traditional past frozen in time, and that as such this constrains and narrows the options for the social practices of indigenous people (Brady 1995). That is, culture has been viewed as something static that needs to be recovered as opposed to something that is dynamic and constantly evolving. There are some parallels here in the cultural revival and nationalism that can be attributed to traditional medicine in the Indian subcontinent.

Traditional healing practices and therapeutic regimens unsurprisingly differed across different first nations and indigenous peoples. In Australia, healing practices were usually private matters commonly involving the 'removal of foreign objects and alien forces from a person' (Bell cited in Brady 1995: 1494) or land-based approaches such as going 'out bush'. By contrast, in North America, therapeutic practices could take the shape of group events and there are differences between, for example, indigenous peoples of the North American plains who have highly ritualised practices and sub-Arctic hunter-gatherers who draw on land-based subsistence activities in therapeutic ways (Brady 1995). But through cross-fertilisation between different First Nations and indigenous groups, there have developed syntheses and hybrid practices in therapeutic approaches, that may also include Western elements (Brady 1995). Programmes can combine elements of First Nations and Western systems, such as the process used by Alcoholics Anonymous and Native American sweat lodges, through to systems based entirely on the medico-religious systems of First Nations (Brady 1995).

Māori health models have been developed in New Zealand with common components including a focus on self-determination, a focus on Māori collective structures such as *whānau* (roughly commensurate with family), *hapū* (a subtribe) and *iwi* (a tribe), promoting Māori identity and promoting social justice (Boulton et al. 2011). Performance indicators to show accountability and monitor achievements in health care have been proposed in New Zealand that attempt to take into account indigenous practices. One such indicator has been to measure activity relating to spiritual health for Māori, which was measured by the involvement of spiritual healers in treatment settings. In particular, it was suggested that the number of traditional healers working with Western practitioners should be assessed (Dew 2003).

These developments in integrating, assimilating or co-opting indigenous medicine indicates a counter current to the dominance of evidence-based medicine. The political and cultural push to recognise First Nations Peoples and their healing practices is not driven by evidence-based medicine and the healing practices are not easily amenable to evidence-based medicine assessments. The drivers of integration are varied and contextually specific, and in this section, the influence of neo-liberalism, corporate capitalism, modernisation and indigenous revitalisation have been discussed.

Communication between modalities

Another level of integration, or lack of it, can be seen in the referral patterns and communication between CAM practitioners and biomedical practitioners who 'share' the same patients. Very often, the biomedical practitioners will not be aware that they are sharing care with a CAM practitioner as neither the patient nor the CAM practitioner is likely to inform the biomedical practitioner about that care (Koenig et al. 2012; Penney et al. 2016). This may be exacerbated if physicians are uncomfortable discussing CAM with their patients, which some research indicates, although this may vary by specialism as most oncology physicians in some research state that they are comfortable talking to their patients about CAM (Roberts et al. 2006).

There are situations where practitioners will know that they are sharing care. Lauren Penney and colleagues discuss the case of a Health Maintenance Organisation in the United States, where nearly all of the 530,000 members have a chiropractic benefit and most have an acupuncture benefit as part of their healthcare plan (Penney et al. 2016). In this case, patients can be referred by primary care physicians to an acupuncturist or chiropractor for a limited number of visits, and this referral must be approved by the Health Maintenance Organisation's referral office. On most occasions, the referral is initiated by the patient, who makes a request for one. GPs respond to this in a number of ways, from assenting through to denying the request. In the study by Penney and colleagues, the primary care physicians would occasionally suggest referral, selecting patients with conditions that they thought might respond well to chiropractic or acupuncture, or because patients had expressed a desire not to use particular drugs recommended. Patient selection could be based on the clinician's assessment of their susceptibility to placebo, as for these clinicians the effectiveness of alternative approaches resulted from the placebo effect. The more common reticence to referral could also be put down to a lack of knowledge that the primary care physicians had of these alternative approaches (Penney et al. 2016).

This lack of knowledge about alternatives is exacerbated by an almost complete absence of communication between the primary care physicians and the acupuncture and chiropractic providers. Some of the physicians would welcome better communication, but others were not sure what it would add. These latter physicians would emphasise the differences of these approaches from Western medicine and so the unlikelihood that the physician could make sense of what alternative practitioners claimed to do.

Any communication that occurred between alternative practitioners and physicians was then left to patients. However, patients were often reluctant to talk to primary care physicians about their alternative treatments, being concerned that such talk would not be well received. There was also a negative bias in reporting, in that patients were more likely to report failures in treatment than successes, as a failure would take them back to the primary care physician whereas success would keep the patient away from said physician. Patients then played a crucial role in negotiating the level of integration and the exchange of knowledge between therapeutic systems, but the level of communication was low, as was the visibility of CAM practices to biomedical practitioners.

Concluding comments

This chapter has explored some of the ways in which we see CAM disciplined and regulated, some as a consequence of developments within biomedicine, such as the rhetorical hegemony of evidence-based medicine, and some specific to CAM, such as the ready uptake of anti-CAM discourses by the media. These mechanisms impact on CAM practices, practitioners, researchers and academics attempting to integrate with statist medicine. CAM coming into the education system is shaped by statist medicine. This shaping can be spurred on by lobbying to maintain (though it has never existed in reality) a pure epistemic culture in state funded education systems. In clinical settings, effort to integrate biomedical and CAM practices may have outcomes of constraining and subordinating CAM. In some settings, efforts at integration may not be so unbalanced, as can be seen in integration developments in China and when indigenous healing practices obtain state support. However, the drivers influencing 'integration' are complex, varied and situationally specific. They can include political and economic factors, cultural revivalism and the actions of citizens. In many instances, it might be more appropriate to speak of assimilation rather than integration. That is, biomedical functionaries selecting aspects of CAM practice that can be incorporated into biomedical understandings. Finally, even with patients' integrating practices, this integration may not be known to biomedical practitioners.

In sum, there are very powerful rhetorical forces, methodological mechanisms and political systems that limit what could be viewed as authentic integration possibilities and limit the possibilities of therapeutic pluralism. In the next chapter, I further explore the disciplining of CAM with the example of chiropractic, and here we will see more fervent efforts to discipline CAM practices, through suppression.

References

Ashmore, M., Mulkay, M. and Pinch, T. (1989) *Health and efficiency: A sociology of health economics*, Milton Keynes: Open University Press.

Baer, H. and Coulter, I. (2008) Taking stock of integrative medicine: Broadening biomedicine or co-option of complementary and alternative medicine?, *Health Sociology Review*, 17, 4, 331–341.

Berg, M. (1997) *Rationalizing medical work: Decision-support techniques and medical practices*, Cambridge: MIT Press.

Boulton, A., Gifford, H., Kauika, A. and Parata, K. (2011) Māori health promotion: Challenges for best practice, *AlterNative: An International Journal of Indigenous Peoples*, 7, 1, 26–39.

Brady, M. (1995) Culture in treatment, culture as treatment: A critical appraisal of developments in addictions programs for indigenous North Americans and Australians, *Social Science & Medicine*, 41, 11, 1487–1498.

Brosnan, C. (2015) 'Quackery' in the academy? Professional knowledge, autonomy and the debate over complementary medicine degrees, *Sociology*, 49, 6, 1047–1064.

——— (2016) Epistemic cultures in complementary medicine: Knowledge-making in university departments of osteopathy and Chinese medicine, *Health Sociology Review*, 25, 2, 171–186.

Cano-Orón, L. (2019) A Twitter campaign against pseudoscience: The sceptical discourse on complementary therapies in Spain, *Public Understanding of Science*, 28, 6, 679–695.

Chamberlain, J.M. (2013) *The sociology of medical regulation: An introduction*, Dordrecht: Springer.

Chamberlain, K., Madden, H., Gabe, J., Dew, K. and Norris, P. (2011) Forms of resistance to medication within New Zealand households, *Medische Anthroplogie*, 23, 2, 299–308.

Checkland, K., Harrison, S., McDonald, R., Grant, S., Campbell, S. and Guthrie, B. (2008) Biomedicine, holism and general medical practice: Responses to the 2004 general practitioner contract, *Sociology of Health & Illness*, 30, 5, 788–803.

Coburn, D., Rappolt, S. and Bourgeault, I. (1997) Decline vs retention of medical power through restratification: An examination of the Ontario case, *Sociology of Health and Illness*, 19, 1–22.

Cochrane, A. (1972) *Effectiveness and efficacy: Random reflections*, London: Nuffield Provincial Hospitals Trust.

Collyer, F. (2004) The corporatisation and commercialisation of CAM, in P. Tovey, G. Easthope and J. Adams (eds.), *The mainstreaming of complementary and alternative medicine: Studies in social context*, London and New York: Routledge, pp. 81–99.

Coulter, I. (2004) Integration and paradigm clash: The practical difficulties of integrative medicine, in P. Tovey, G. Easthope and J. Adams (eds.), *The mainstreaming of complementary and alternative medicine: Studies in social context*, London: Routledge, pp. 103–122.

Dew, K. (2000) Deviant insiders: Medical acupuncturists in New Zealand, *Social Science & Medicine*, 50, 12, 1785–1795.

——— (2003) *Borderland practices: Regulating alternative therapies in New Zealand*, Dunedin: University of Otago Press.

Dew, K., Chamberlain, K., Hodgetts, D., Norris, P., Radley, A. and Gabe, J. (2014) Home as a hybrid centre of medication practice, *Sociology of Health & Illness*, 36, 1, 28–43.

Ellis, R. and Whittington, D. (1993) *Quality assurance in health care: A handbook*, London: Edward Arnold.

Frenk, J. and Durán-Arenas, I. (1993) The medical profession and the state, in F. Hafferty and J. McKinlay (eds.), *The changing medical profession: An international perspective*, New York: Oxford University Press, pp. 25–42.

Fries, C.J. (2008) Governing the health of the hybrid self: Integrative medicine, neoliberalism, and the shifting biopolitics of subjectivity, *Health Sociology Review*, 17, 4, 353–367.

Green, J. (2000) Epistemology, evidence and experience: Evidence based health care in the work of accident alliances, *Sociology of Health & Illness*, 22, 4, 453–476.

Hacking, I. (1990) *The taming of chance*, Cambridge: Cambridge University Press.

Hess, D.J. (2004) Medical modernisation, scientific research fields and the epistemic politics of health social movements, *Sociology of Health & Illness*, 26, 6, 695–709.

Hollenberg, D. and Muzzin, L. (2010) Epistemological challenges to integrative medicine: An anti-colonial perspective on the combination of complementary/alternative medicine with biomedicine, *Health Sociology Review*, 19, 1, 34–56.

Jackson, S. and Scambler, G. (2007) Perceptions of evidence-based medicine: Traditional acupuncturists in the UK and resistance to biomedical modes of evaluation, *Sociology of Health & Illness*, 29, 3, 412–429.

Janes, C. (2002) Buddhism, science, and market: The globalisation of Tibetan medicine, *Anthropology & Medicine*, 9, 3, 267–289.

Jost, T.S. (1992) Recent developments in medical quality assurance and audit, in R. Dingwall and P. Fenn (eds.), *Quality and regulation in health care: International experiences*, London: Routledge, pp. 69–88.

Koenig, C.J., Ho, E.Y., Yadegar, V. and Tarn, D.M. (2012) Negotiating complementary and alternative medicine use in primary care visits with older patients, *Patient Education and Counseling*, 89, 3, 368–373.

Langford, J. (2002) *Fluent bodies: Ayurvedic remedies for postcolonial imbalance*, Durham: Duke University Press.

Lewis, M. (2019) De-legitimising complementary medicine: Framings of the friends of science in medicine-CAM debate in Australian media reports, *Sociology of Health & Illness*, 41, 5, 831–851.

Light, D. (2010) The Food and Drug Administration: Inadequate protection from serious risks, in D. Light (ed.), *The risks of prescription drugs*, New York: Columbia University Press, pp. 40–68.

Lipman, T. (2000) Power and influence in clinical effectiveness and evidence-based medicine, *Family Practice*, 17, 6, 557–563.

Marmor, T.R., Barer, M.L. and Evans, R.G. (1994) The determinants of a population's health: What can be done to improve a democratic nation's health status?, in R.G. Evans, M.L. Barer and T.R. Marmor (eds.), *Why are some people healthy and others not? The determinants of health of populations*, New York: Aldine De Gruyter, pp. 217–230.

Maynard, A. (1995) Distributing health care rationing and the role of the physician in the United Kingdom National Health Service, in A. Grubb and M.J. Mehlman (eds.), *Justice and health care: Comparative perspectives*, Chichester: John Wiley and Sons, pp. 305–321.

Mizrachi, N., Shuval, J.T. and Gross, S. (2005) Boundary at work: Alternative medicine in biomedical settings, *Sociology of Health & Illness*, 27, 1, 20–43.

Murard, L. (2008) Designs within disorder: International conferences on rural health care and the art of the local, 1931–39, in S. Gross Solomon, L. Murard and P. Zylberman (eds.), *Shifting boundaries of public health: Europe in the twentieth century*, Rochester: University of Rochester Press, pp. 141–174.

Pearson, D. (2001) *The politics of ethnicity in settler societies: States of unease*, Houndmills: Palgrave.

Penney, L.S., Ritenbaugh, C., Elder, C., Schneider, J., Deyo, R.A. and Debar, L.L. (2016) Primary care physicians, acupuncture and chiropractic clinicians, and chronic pain patients: A qualitative analysis of communication and care coordination patterns, *BMC Complementary and Alternative Medicine*, 16, 29, 30.

Porter, R. (2006) Medical science, in R. Porter (ed.), *The Cambridge history of medicine*, Cambridge: Cambridge University Press, pp. 136–175.

Porter, T. (1995) *Trust in numbers: The pursuit of objectivity in science and public life*, Princeton: Princeton University Press.

Possamai-Inesedy, A. and Cochrane, S. (2013) The consequences of integrating complementary and alternative medicine: An analysis of impacts on practice, *Health Sociology Review*, 22, 1, 65–74.

Roberts, C.S., Baker, F., Hann, D., Runfola, J., Witt, C., McDonald, J., Livingston, M.L., Ruiterman, J., Ampela, R., Kaw, O.C. and Blanchard, C. (2006) Patient-physician communication regarding use of complementary therapies during cancer treatment, *Journal of Psychosocial Oncology*, 23, 4, 35–60.

Scheid, V. (2002) *Chinese medicine in contemporary China: Plurality and synthesis*, Durham, NC: Duke University Press.

Seale, C. (1993) The consumer voice, in B. Davey and J. Popay (eds.), *Dilemmas in health care*, Buckingham: Open University Press, pp. 64–80.

Seedhouse, D. (1995) The way around health economics' dead end, *Health Care Analysis*, 3, 205–220.

Sharp, D., Lorenc, A., Little, P., Mercer, S.W., Hollinghurst, S., Feder, G. and MacPherson, H. (2018) Complementary medicine and the NHS: Experiences of integration with UK primary care, *European Journal of Integrative Medicine*, 24, 8–16.

Singer, J. and Fisher, K. (2007) The impact of co-option on herbalism: A bifurcation in epistemology and practice, *Health Sociology Review*, 16, 1, 18–26.

Tenbensel, T. (2000) Health prioritisation as rationalist policy making: Problems, prognoses and prospects, *Policy and Politics*, 28, 3, 425–440.

4

ADJUSTING TO STATIST MEDICINE AND THE MANIPULATION OF CHIROPRACTIC

Chiropractors are usually associated with the treatment of bad backs, but in its original conception chiropractic had a much wider scope of practice. Chiropractic began in 1895 when D. D. Palmer performed the first chiropractic spinal adjustment. Palmer claimed that his janitor had put his back out seventeen years earlier, and since that time, he had been deaf. Palmer adjusted a misplaced vertebra and the janitor immediately recovered his hearing. Palmer went on to manipulate the backs of other people with a variety of ailments. He believed that disease results from subluxations of spinal vertebrae, with the subluxation interfering with the transmission of neural impulses and through that mechanism causing disease. Manipulation of the misplaced vertebra is famously achieved by the chiropractic thrust to said vertebra (Smith-Cunnien 1998).

Chiropractic was not founded as a treatment for bad backs, but for other conditions that might be related to the spine, and coincidentally also related to bad backs. The original philosophy of chiropractic suggested that many diseases were caused by interference with the nerves as they passed out of the spinal column. Removing subluxations restored the flow of the innate intelligence of the body. Such claims situate chiropractic as a vitalist therapeutic approach and as alternative to biomedicine (Brosnan 2017). However, chiropractic has struggled to gain legitimacy for its claims, and it has frequently conflicted with biomedicine. The conflict has limited the claims made by chiropractors, and by implication limited its practice, and so the example of chiropractic illustrates one way in which therapeutic pluralism is contained by biomedicine and statist medicine. This chapter explores struggles over chiropractic's claims about its scope of practice, arguing that the scope of chiropractic therapeutic practice has become limited, which is at least in part an outcome of the struggles chiropractic has had with orthodox medicine, which strenuously opposed any notion that chiropractors could treat organic diseases.

Early struggles

Chiropractic is a therapeutic approach that could be considered indigenous to the United States. It is not the only approach. Christian Science, Thomsonism (a botanically based modality) and closer to chiropractic, osteopathy, are all developments within the borders of the United States, and there are many others. I was trained as an osteopath in the United Kingdom, and osteopathy shares with chiropractic the use of different forms of spinal manipulation to enhance health. When I was asked what is the difference between chiropractic and osteopathy I sometimes jokingly told an apocryphal story that D. D. Palmer attended the first osteopathic school, founded in 1892, for one month then left to establish chiropractic in 1895, so chiropractic insights are one month's worth of osteopathy. No doubt chiropractic students are told similar apocryphal stories about osteopathy. This story suggests the kind of rivalry that can occur between alternative therapies, further contesting the view that we can treat them homogenously.

In alignment with professionalising strategies of occupational groups, chiropractors formed professional associations in the early stages of its existence, and established educational facilities, patient support groups and also lobbied for legislative recognition (Baer 2001). However, from the early days of chiropractic, there were different factions or different epistemic cultures within its ranks. That is, as noted in Chapter 3, factions with different values, practices and understandings. The factions were named 'straights' and 'mixers', with the straights limiting chiropractic to spinal adjustment and the mixers incorporating other therapeutic elements such as diet, exercise and hydropathy (Baer 2001). Hydropathy, or hydrotherapy, has a long history as a therapeutic approach and can extend from ingesting water to bathing and saunas, cold water being poured over the body and cold sheets being wrapped around the patient. These factions formed their own associations and training establishments. By the 1980s, chiropractic had established a united front in efforts to gain a better footing in the healthcare system, including Medicare in the United States (Baer 2001). Medicare is a national health insurance scheme that mainly provides cover for those over 65.

Although chiropractic positioned itself as a complete healing system efforts to achieve this were short lived as the cost of establishing and operating hospitals with comprehensive care facilities was untenable, particularly with an absence of government funding and third-party pay outs (Baer 2001). Most chiropractic treatments then focus on musculo-skeletal concerns (Baer 2001). The requirements to attain what is expected of a complete healing system were not then achievable without high levels of state support. Chiropractic was not able to become a functionary of state medicine, although it was able to obtain lesser levels of state support.

Chiropractors were successful at gaining state licensing laws in some states from the early twentieth century although the last state to do so, Mississippi, held out until 1973. The scope of practice however varied significantly across states from those that only allowed for spinal adjustment to those that extended out to such items as the performance of minor surgery and the signing of birth and death certificates (Baer 2001). A cost of licensure for chiropractors is that in order to pass licensing examinations chiropractic colleges had to adjust their curricula, so that the colleges more closely resembled biomedical schools (Baer 2001). Chiropractic could then make gains in terms of state recognition, but at a cost of conforming more closely to the biomedical paradigm.

Efforts to suppress chiropractic in its place of birth were intense. In the early years of chiropractic, medical physicians would enrol law enforcement agencies to prosecute chiropractors for practicing without a license (Baer 2001). After the first World War, the American Medical Association intensified efforts to suppress chiropractic, including lobbying efforts to prevent chiropractic patients accessing Medicare and other insurance cover and preventing American Medical Association members from associating with or referring patients to chiropractors (Baer 2001).

Chester Wilks and four other chiropractors brought an antitrust suit against the American Medical Association in the 1980s. The Wilks vs American Medical Association judgment found against the American Medical Association, finding it guilty of restricting trade and conspiring to eliminate chiropractic (Baer and Coulter 2008). Prior to the start of this trial, the American Medical Association had an ethical ruling precluding Association members from professionally associating with anyone who violated the principle that healing was founded on a scientific basis. This meant in practice that members were not allowed to associate with chiropractors, but the American Medical Association rescinded this ruling in 1978. However, following the loss of this suit, the American Medical Association still continued to attack chiropractic (Baer 2001).

Despite the efforts to undermine chiropractic, it has persisted. Other research suggests that chiropractic's survival in the face of medical opposition has been due to a number of influences, such as popular demand for its services, aggressive lobbying of legislators and the state becoming increasingly involved in the organisation of health services (Clavarino and Yates 1995; Coburn and Biggs 1986; Smith-Cunnien 1998; Willis 1983). Hans Baer argues that chiropractic offered a path to the American dream for the working class and the lower middle-class who were usually blocked from careers in biomedicine as a result of structural barriers, such as access to resources and quality education outcomes (Baer 2001).

The next sections of this chapter will turn to a particular public hearing on chiropractic. A focus on this hearing allows for a close examination of the rhetorical and discursive strategies deployed by both the profession of chiropractic and its opponents. By understanding the argumentation that is made, we get a sense of important mechanisms that limit the possibilities of therapeutic pluralism in Western countries. The detailed case study of a Commission of Inquiry into Chiropractic that follows provides an in-depth understanding of more general processes that shape not only the therapeutic possibilities of chiropractic, but of any professional body that poses a challenge to biomedicine.

Public hearings

In New Zealand, chiropractic has doggedly struggled to be included in the public health system. The pivotal event for chiropractic was the 1978 Commission of Inquiry into Chiropractic. This Inquiry was a rare event in the history of relations between alternative medicine and orthodox medicine, in that the opposing sides came together to present their cases in the presence of 'impartial' judges. The Commission of Inquiry into Chiropractic started its hearings in May 1978, completing its final report in September 1979. In making their recommendations, the Commission was to consider the scientific and educational basis of chiropractic, and whether it constitutes a distinct healing art (Dew 2000). By examining this event, we witness the disputes between the two factions, medicine and chiropractic, and see how the Commissioners resolved these seemingly incompatible positions. The way in which this impartial body resolved these opposites reveals key forces at work in disputes over the validation of knowledge claims and this in turn links to claims about what can be practiced by different healers. The way in which the recommendations of the Commissioners became altered when acted upon by the state demonstrates the constraints on alternative health practises imposed by the power of the medical profession as a functionary of statist medicine.

The resolution of this struggle between chiropractic and the medical establishment occurred, in part, through a process of chiropractic redefining itself and limiting the claims it made about what the therapy could do. It did this in order to allow for a 'workable' relationship within the structure of health service delivery. In turn, the medical profession re-positioned itself in relation to alternative therapies, moving from a situation where medical practitioners were not allowed to have any professional relationship with chiropractors, to one where they could refer patients to chiropractors for treatment. Considering these debates gives insight into the intricacies of the process of negotiation and to the series of tensions that chiropractic had to reconcile. It also provides an opportunity to appraise the normative system of medicine and to discern ways in which a new set of norms evolves. An examination of this controversy allows us to understand how incompatible systems become compatible and the evolving nature of orthodoxy and heterodoxy, and gives an indication of the balancing act that alternative practitioners are required to perform when arguing for greater legitimacy in an open forum, whilst simultaneously having to argue that a working relationship can be developed between themselves and their 'enemies'. Since the Inquiry in 1978, there have been movements within the medical profession towards evidence-based medicine, discussed in Chapter 3, that have altered the way in which alternative modalities present themselves before legislative bodies.

In the Commission of Inquiry into Chiropractic (1979), there were 136 formal submissions made to the Commission, coming to more than 2,300 pages. Oral evidence amounted to 3,658 pages of transcript presented over a period of seventy-eight days. In addition, the Commission received nearly 13,000 completed questionnaire forms from chiropractic patients. The New Zealand Chiropractors' Association had printed these forms and encouraged chiropractic patients to complete them and send them in to the Commission. The Commission visited the medical schools at Otago and Auckland and the schools of physiotherapy in Auckland and Dunedin in New Zealand. In addition, chiropractic colleges were inspected in Australia, England, Canada and the United States.

The accounts of the scientific enterprise given by the representatives of established medicine, and the chiropractors' accounts of their achievements that we see in these debates, are reifying discourses. A reifying discourse is where something abstract is turned into a material thing, where an event, a thought or a set of circumstances, is produced as an object (Potter 1996). The medical view that the chiropractic subluxation is simply standard degenerative disease in the spine is one example. Ironising discourses are also used in these debates, where the literal descriptiveness of versions is undermined, where 'the material thing (is turned) back into talk which is motivated, distorted or erroneous in some way' (Potter 1996: 107). In this Inquiry, we see the medical practitioners positioning chiropractors as motivated by such things as 'salesmanship', whereas the chiropractors charge the medical groups with being motivated by the desire to protect their monopoly.

In addition to reifying and ironising discourses, this case study demonstrates another important discourse in public confrontations between orthodox and alternative medicine. It is suggested here that the chiropractors had to employ a de-reifying or esoteric discourse. This was necessary, as chiropractors had to resist a description of their activities in purely medical terms. If the medical establishment successfully employed a reifying discourse to describe chiropractic in medical terms, then there would in effect be no need for a separate occupational grouping of chiropractors outside of medical control.

Accounts provided by participants in this Inquiry can be viewed as having a double orientation. Accounts have an epistemological orientation, attempting to establish their own status as factual. Accounts also have an action orientation in that they are used to accomplish some action (Potter 1996). The protagonists can be seen as uncompromising in terms of their epistemological orientation, but the action orientation of accounts allows for more manoeuvres on the part of both sides. The Royal Commission of Inquiry in turn tempered these accounts, leading to a version of the world different from that of the two protagonists. This new account was further mediated by the state, leading to actions or arrangements that were not necessarily envisaged by the Commission. Here, we have a translation of these accounts to workable practices, where incompatible systems become compatible with the paradigm of statist medicine.

This Inquiry was important for the chiropractic profession in New Zealand as, prior to it, few chiropractic patients could benefit from the New Zealand accident compensation system run by the Accident Compensation Corporation that was established in 1974. Since 1974, the country had a no-fault response to adverse events associated with injuries. The scheme would bring to an end the frequently disappointing process of common law action based upon negligence, which produced widely varying outcomes for people suffering the same injuries. Patients who were eligible for compensation could have all or most of their treatment costs funded by the Accident Compensation Corporation. However, under Accident Compensation Corporation rules when it was established, a patient could only gain eligibility for chiropractic treatment if a medical practitioner had made a referral. Such referrals were very rare.

In 1975, a petition was presented to the New Zealand parliament to allow chiropractic patients to be compensated for the cost of chiropractic treatment in cases of personal injury. Following this petition, in 1978, it was recorded in the Medical Association's handbook that 'it is unethical for a doctor to refer a patient to a chiropractor for treatment' (Commission of Inquiry into Chiropractic 1979: 255). In this, the New Zealand Medical Association used the same tactics as the American Medical Association in trying to undermine chiropractic. As chiropractic services could only be compensated for if a medical practitioner recommended those services, it was now impossible for doctors to make such referrals.

The submissions to the inquiry that took place in 1978 polarised into two camps. On the one side, there was the medical profession and its allies: the physiotherapists, the Department of Health and the New Zealand Consumer Council. On the other were the chiropractors and their allies – the thousands of patients who sent in letters and survey forms expounding the virtues of chiropractic, and groups representing workers, such as the Federation of Labour.

Some features of the debates that occurred at the Inquiry have been noted in other studies. Chiropractors were criticised for their lack of training, particularly as they acted as a first point of contact for patients. This issue was also a concern in Australia and Canada when chiropractors were seeking greater legitimacy (Willis 1983, Coburn and Biggs 1986). The medical profession argued that the systems of medicine and chiropractic were incompatible, and that as chiropractic was an unproven treatment directed at an unlimited range of disorders it would be absurd for chiropractic to be recognised by the state. Chiropractors responded to the issue of training by suggesting that medically trained manipulators were inadequately trained, and that chiropractic training programmes were the only ones 'designed to prepare the graduates adequately to practice manipulative therapy as primary contact practitioners' (all quotes are taken from submissions to the inquiry). The medical profession also attacked chiropractic for creating unnecessary markets through their family plans that would 'induce an undesirable level of hypochondria in the community'. Chiropractors defended themselves against such attacks by claiming that they would save the state money by reducing spending on pharmaceuticals and returning people quickly to productive work (Dew 2000).

The debates before the Commission also support Evan Willis's view that the medical profession demand scientific legitimacy for chiropractic, whilst chiropractors offered clinical legitimacy (Willis 1983). The latter was found in the popular support chiropractic gained. Social scientists were called in to defend the medical profession. John McKinlay, the professor of sociology at Boston University, argued that submissions from patients were worthless in assessing effectiveness because they were opinion. The New Zealand Chiropractors' Association responded by arguing that the effectiveness of chiropractic was demonstrated as it was supported by the public despite its competitive disadvantages.

The medical profession suggested that if chiropractors were accorded acceptance then the same privileges will be demanded by many other fringe systems of medical care, such as faith healers, naturopaths and colour therapists. This is the 'thin end of the wedge' argument, where there is a concern over where to draw the line if chiropractors are recognised and how to exclude others who claim to supply some form of treatment.

The above provides a brief outline of the core arguments made by both sides in the Inquiry. However, in order to gain insight into the very tricky process of negotiation performed by the chiropractors, some specific strategies are worth dwelling on. I have termed these 'no limits to treatment', 'establishing distinctiveness', 'de-radicalising' and 'indeterminacy' strategies (Dew 2000).

No limits to treatment

Chiropractors were accused of claiming to 'cure everything from pimples to polio', implying that chiropractors are dangerous and irrational practitioners because they did not stick to simple musculo-skeletal conditions, and that they did not place limits on what they would treat. The Medical Association argued that chiropractors 'considered it within their scope of practice the treatment of such diverse conditions as hypertension, whooping cough and diabetes'. Chiropractors were portrayed as posing a danger to the health of their patients, particularly the risk of postponing proper medical care. As some overseas chiropractors had denounced vaccinations, chiropractors in general posed a public health threat if they were given any credibility. If chiropractors do not support vaccinations, then little more needed to be said to indicate their irrationality.

The Chiropractors' Association responded by providing a definition of chiropractic that made no testable therapeutic claims:

> Chiropractic is that science and art which utilizes the inherent recuperative powers of the body and deals with the relationship between the nervous system and the spinal column, including the immediate articulations and the role of this relationship in the restoration and maintenance of health.

In this definition, the Chiropractors' Association avoided making claims about treating any particular condition but proffered a general approach to all conditions. This lack of specificity in the claim implied that there was no limitation to what could be treated but it avoided confrontations over specific claims. The chiropractors had to balance opposing forces here. On the one hand, they had to present themselves as alternative enough from medical practitioners to warrant recognition, but on the other hand, they had to dissociate themselves from claims that might appear irrational.

Establish distinctiveness

Submissions by physiotherapists argued that chiropractors could contribute to New Zealand health services if they developed their standards to that of the Medical Council, practised physical therapy to the standard of the New Zealand Physiotherapy Board, dissociated from the terms chiropractor and chiropractic, and confined their treatments to conditions indicated by science as being amenable to manipulative therapy. In other words, chiropractic could contribute to New Zealand health services if chiropractors gave up their control over their own standards and if they lost their identity as a distinct group.

Chiropractors had to then deploy a rhetorical strategy of establishing distinctiveness in order to claim a special place in healthcare delivery. The Chiropractors' Association used technical language in order to claim distinctiveness from other health practitioners who used spinal manipulation.

> Where is the doctor of medicine or physiotherapist who, when confronted with a lumbar intervertebral disc syndrome and contemplating making a Chiropractic adjustment in treatment, can evaluate the comparative worth's of the Cox chiro-manis technique, the sacro-occipital technique, the Gonstead disc technique, and the Reinert technique, and proceed accordingly?

The chiropractors here attempt to distinguish what they do from what anyone else does and illustrate their own expertise by appealing to specific, named techniques that had been developed within chiropractic. Whilst chiropractors made themselves distinct, but not too distinct, the medical profession alternated between portraying chiropractic as an extreme alternative philosophy, to portraying it as a limited sub-speciality with no distinct features except its misguided philosophy.

De-radicalising

Another strategy adopted by chiropractors was to de-radicalise their philosophy and claims in order to make them more acceptable, and to show themselves as progressive. They argued that the education of chiropractors followed that of other health professionals and had a foundation in basic science. The Chiropractors' Association distanced itself from the views of the founders of chiropractic and some current practitioners by denying that chiropractors believed in one cause for all disease, suggesting instead that chiropractic was a speciality. They submitted that much of the antagonism towards chiropractic was due to the philosophy propounded by Palmer, the founder of chiropractic, that 'a subluxated vertebra is the cause of ninety-five percent of all diseases'. This criticism, according to the submission, ignored the fact that medicine had strange unsupportable ideas at the time of Palmer's discovery, and that chiropractic 'has developed and advanced to an astonishing degree' since Palmer's time.

It was also argued in chiropractic submissions that the clinical evidence on spinal manipulation influencing internal organ function, the most controversial claim of chiropractors, 'is sketchy and based primarily on anecdotal reporting and opinion originating from individual experience together with the occasional uncontrolled trial' and that the link was only a possibility. This statement positions chiropractic in a framework acceptable to a biomedical scientific sensibility, one that the Commissioners found persuasive. The sketchy nature of the evidence about influence on internal organs and its anecdotal nature are the same sorts of criticisms that the medical profession levelled at chiropractic in general. This is an effort to 'de-controversialise' chiropractic, and in doing so move it towards a position that would be found acceptable to the medical establishment.

The abandonment of what some might have seen as the central tenets of chiropractic philosophy became an important feature in the gaining of credibility for that profession. The scientific evidence was debatable in the case of chiropractic improving back pain, as it was in chiropractic improving asthma, but the medical profession would not brook, under any circumstances, the possibility of the latter. This categorised chiropractic as a speciality as opposed to the claim that it was an alternative healing system. In this instance, chiropractors are defining themselves as functioning in the limited field of spinal manipulation and so are posing no threat to GPs. Yet at the same time, the Chiropractors' Association did not want to place limits around what this speciality could do. They argued that 'Chiropractors do not contend that subluxation, however defined, is the most significant causal factor in disease' but suggested that 'in the current state of knowledge it is both unscientific and meaningless to endeavour to limit the range of conditions amenable to Chiropractic therapy'. However, the Chiropractors' Association distanced itself from the more radical claims of its founder, in particular that the 'subluxation' was responsible for most diseases. But they attempted to prevent the limitation of chiropractic to simply dealing with back problems, by appealing to a lack in the current state of knowledge, therefore creating the space for chiropractors to treat a wider range of conditions. There was a continuous wavering between these positions, from chiropractic as a 'healing system' to chiropractic as a specialised form of spinal manipulation.

Medical submissions also attempted to de-radicalise chiropractic. The physiotherapists stated that:

> Chiropractic, it is now trite to say, has no corner on manipulative therapy, and osteopathy for example had already preceded chiropractic down the historical road. Osteopathy began with the cultist belief in the universal value of manipulative therapy. After having adopted the scientific method,

> osteopathy has finished up with practices virtually indistinguishable from allopathic medicine – and so it must be with chiropractic.

The physiotherapists are suggesting that the development of osteopathy in the United States is the pattern for the development of other therapies that attempt to gain wider legitimacy. It implies a linear development from cultist belief to the inevitable acceptance of the principles and practices of orthodox medicine, of the one truth. This triumph of truth is further expressed by the physiotherapists when they state that:

> Anybody with an understanding of the natural sciences must admit that there is only one reality and anyone conducting basic research will discover the same reality as others have.

This is a direct attack on the 'esoteric' nature of the chiropractic notion of the subluxation and the role of manipulation in alleviating disease.

Indeterminacy

The chiropractors had to balance between de-radicalising their claims and keeping themselves clearly distinct from the medical profession and other health professionals. The medical profession also engaged in de-radicalising the claims of chiropractic relating chiropractic's seemingly esoteric claims about subluxations to more mundane matters. Employing a reifying discourse, the New Zealand Medical Association submitted that the chiropractic subluxation was 'an ordinary sign of degenerative spinal disease' familiar to orthodox doctors. Yet chiropractors made the claim that a subluxated vertebra disturbed the nerve supply of an organ that ultimately caused pathology.

The claim that a subluxation could cause organ pathology and disease was untenable to the medical profession. For them, the subluxation is made into something familiar and insignificant. On the other hand, chiropractors posited a hierarchy of skills, with the highest rung only being attained by the dedicated chiropractor:

> The physical application of the Chiropractic adjustment is largely a mechanical skill the fundamentals of which may be mastered over some months. To acquire the specialised palpating skills basic to Chiropractic diagnosis is more difficult. However, complicated factors of physiology and philosophical understanding involved in the basic evaluation of the patient are infinitely more important and exacting and serve to explain why Chiropractic has remained a separate and distinct science and why many patients respond to Chiropractic following failure under other therapies.

The term chiropractic adjustment used in this quote can be read as a substitute for the term spinal manipulation, something potentially carried out by medical manipulators, physiotherapists with an interest in that area and practitioners beyond statist medicine such as osteopaths. The connotation is that this aspect of chiropractic is easily learnt. But the higher levels of expertise are not so easily learnt. To achieve chiropractic diagnostic capabilities, which implies detecting subluxations, special palpation skills are required. The subluxation here is not simply spinal degeneration that can be identified by X-rays, but a specific functional impairment of spinal movement. Finally, reference to physiology and philosophy suggests that we are now in the domain that only fully trained chiropractors can access.

Expertise is based on a notion of philosophical understanding, a contrast with the simple mechanics of spinal manipulation. The chiropractors employ an esoteric discourse to argue that the art and science of chiropractic has a high indeterminacy/technicality ratio (Jamous and Peloille 1970). A high indeterminacy/technicality ratio provides a protective barrier for the medical profession. The profession lays claim to a high level of technicality and therefore has a grounding in the scientific disciplines, but also fosters a mystique of indeterminate knowledge so their field of activity cannot be reduced to routine, and so it can resist a downgrading of its status (Turner 1987). According to Paul Atkinson (1997: 6), it is knowledge that is defined as indeterminate, a knowledge which 'is not susceptible to rational codification and explicit statement'. As Atkinson (1997: 184) suggests, 'the notions of indetermination and technicality constitute a rhetoric in which are couched claims concerning professional work and expertise'. The chiropractors attempted to build a barrier to codification by emphasising esoteric aspects of their practice beyond the relatively simple skills of spinal manipulation, and in addition provided a rhetorical response to the reifying discourse of the medical profession.

Findings and outcomes

The chiropractors closing submission concluded with recommendations that chiropractors should be able to write certificates that would allow chiropractic patients to receive payments from the Accident Compensation Corporation and the sickness benefit; that the medical association ethical ruling be rescinded; that tertiary benefits be payable for approved chiropractic colleges; that the practice of spinal manipulation be restricted to chiropractors, specialist medical practitioners and those medical practitioners and physiotherapists who had passed a course in spinal manipulative therapy as prescribed by the Chiropractic Board, and anyone else the board approved of; that chiropractors should not be excluded from hospitals. The Commissioners agreed on all counts.

The imagery presented by the protagonists in this debate appears to be alarmingly simple, and surprisingly black and white, yet the arguments were flexible, complex and at times inconsistent. For the medical profession, the chiropractors were health frauds, deceiving the public and marketing their swindling services in sophisticated ways. The patients were dupes, unable to distinguish between placebo and cure, taken in by the salesman's charm of the chiropractor. Chiropractors held to a ridiculous philosophy that had no basis in science, and scientifically trained medical practitioners should have nothing to do with chiropractors. If they were genuinely concerned with healing then let them become medical practitioners and train in the same way that medical practitioners do.

For the chiropractors, the medical profession was a unified monopoly protecting its turf. It was arrogant and overbearing and would go to any ends to defeat its enemy, no matter how small and insignificant that enemy was. The medical profession was only concerned for itself and had no interest in the health of the population. If it had it would have tried to understand why chiropractic was so successful.

At the conclusion of the Inquiry, the Commissioners levelled a number of criticisms at the medical profession and rejected the case that it made. The Commissioners found that chiropractors were the only health practitioners who were necessarily equipped by their education and training to carry out spinal manual therapy for which general medical practitioners and physiotherapists had no adequate training. It recommended that chiropractic gain access to state health benefits that were available to medical doctors for the treatment of back problems.

The strategy adopted by the Commissioners to reconcile competing claims was to situate chiropractic firmly within a paradigm of science that was acceptable to medicine. In doing so, it supported the training of chiropractors but limited its claims about treating organic disease and the interpretations that could be placed on its philosophy. The Commissioners dismissed criticisms of chiropractic education and training, arguing that chiropractic used medical and scientific knowledge as its foundation, and where this was inconclusive, they relied on clinical experience, but that there was nothing in chiropractic that was 'radically inconsistent with a scientific approach'.

In relation to medical standards of spinal therapy, the Commissioners suggested that medical practitioners would need at least a year's full-time training to reach the standards of a qualified chiropractor. The Commissioners were critical of medical practitioners using manual therapy, arguing that 'what evidence we have received is largely that of patients whose experience of attempts at manual therapy by their own doctor drove them to a chiropractor'. Due to the specialised nature of spinal manual therapy, it was noted that chiropractors should be responsible for training and part-time courses for other health professionals should be discouraged.

The Commissioners concluded that government funding for manipulative therapy education should be better allocated to enable physiotherapists to attend chiropractic colleges. Physiotherapists, who bitterly opposed chiropractic, now had the prospect of having to enter the institutions of their enemies and be subjected to what they would consider as chiropractic's untenable teachings. The Commissioners rejected the view that patient support for chiropractic was anecdotal or mere opinion. Those who had appeared before the Commission who had experience of chiropractic treatment vividly conveyed the difference that chiropractic treatment had made to their lives. The Commissioners were sympathetic to chiropractic claims without being convinced of their philosophical underpinnings. They suggested that 'chiropractic is a form of treatment still in search of an explanation for its effectiveness' (Commission of Inquiry into Chiropractic 1979: 44). They argued that the subluxation was a functional abnormality that could be identified by those with the specialised skills and training of chiropractors. Chiropractors could also relieve conditions, or at least back pain, caused by the subluxation. In this, the Commissioners accepted the indeterminacy of chiropractic practice and its esoteric discourse, that there was such a thing as a subluxation, that it at least could be the cause of back pain and that chiropractors could detect it and treat it.

Despite the overwhelming support for chiropractic, the Commissioners were not prepared to give chiropractors the prestige and privilege of the medical profession. The Commissioners suggested that chiropractors should have limited their attention to 'cases of backache' and because they did not do this and because some chiropractors tried to persuade their patients to consult them before their doctor, this 'antagonised the organised medical profession' (Commission of Inquiry into Chiropractic 1979: 27). The Commissioners were critical of the chiropractic profession for failing to define their scope of practice. In effect, the Commissioners were denying chiropractic the position of being an alternative form of therapy but positioned chiropractic as offering services complementary to the medical profession. The Commissioners suggested that chiropractic techniques were not very different from those of others who specialised in manual therapy, and that it would be wrong to treat chiropractic as a healing art separate from orthodox medicine. Additionally, they accepted the medical position that 'the only person qualified to carry out a proper differential diagnosis is a medical practitioner'.

The Commissioners rejected the Chiropractors' Association's view that chiropractic was a separate and distinct healing art, stating that it is no more separate than 'dentistry, psychiatry, physiotherapy or any other speciality'. However, the Commissioners were of the view that chiropractic was an independent profession, and not in the position of a medical auxiliary to a medical practitioner, as in the case of physiotherapy.

The findings of the Commission were perceived as a great victory for chiropractic, but that victory came at a cost. In order to become acceptable, the chiropractors had to pose no threat to the niche occupied by most GPs, all of who could potentially refer patients to them. The president of the New Zealand Chiropractors' Association went so far as to state in 1991 that 'chiropractic does not seek to treat disease by manipulation', but their 'central interest has always been the impaired movement of vertebrae' and 'in the last ten years the profession has established . . . a new era of cooperation with medicine' (Stinear 1991). This limitation of chiropractic has been commented on by other authors in different countries. Saks (1994) argues that alternative practitioners in Britain frequently dilute the radicalism of their ideas. Coburn notes a similar 'de-radicalising' occurring in Canada where some provinces have given official recognition to chiropractic as a self-governing health occupation but at the expense of narrowing the scope of what can be practised. Coburn (1993) goes so far as to say that chiropractic has been tamed and medicalised. Similar arguments have been made about chiropractors in Australia (Clavarino and Yates 1995; Willis 1983).

The medical profession is not a static entity, and its boundaries are changing constantly. An important concept in these boundary changes is that of professional self-interest (Saks 1992). Saks argues that the medical profession will either accept or reject therapeutic techniques and methods of diagnosis depending on the strategy from which it will derive the most benefit. Over time different strategies may be employed. Saks shows this in Britain with acupuncturists, and the same strategy can be seen in New Zealand with chiropractic. This ability to change strategies can be seen in the haste with which the Medical Association changed its code of ethics. In 1978, it was unethical for doctors to refer patients to chiropractors but faced with the possibility of chiropractors being able to see Accident Compensation Corporation patients without a medical referral this ruling was dropped in 1980. In doing so, the medical profession retained greater control over the chiropractic profession.

This case shows how an apparently successful outcome for a previously invalidated therapy may lead to greater levels of limitation and regulation of that therapy. The debate before an impartial tribunal concluded with the medical profession being criticised for its stance. We rarely see such searing criticisms being made of the medical profession in relation to alternative therapies. This case also shows the problems that any alternative therapy faces in achieving a balance between remaining distinctive and de-radicalising. One strategy to resolve this is to highlight the indeterminacy and esoteric nature of the therapeutic practice. This strategy gave the Commissioners an important link in its attempt to re-negotiate the relationship between medicine and chiropractic.

Although the Inquiry led to the dropping of the medical profession's ethical clause preventing referrals by doctors to chiropractors, it appears to have done little else for chiropractors. Chiropractors do not oversee the education of spinal manipulation in New Zealand, and they will not be found working in the hospital system. In arguing for greater legitimacy in an open forum, whilst simultaneously having to argue that a working relationship can be developed between them and their opponents, chiropractors were ultimately drawn into a subordinate relationship with medicine. The attempt to remain distinctive, but not hold on to an incommensurable position broke down as chiropractic was located by the Commission within an orthodox epistemological position. Yet at the same time, the Commission recommended wide-ranging changes to the relationship between orthodox medicine and chiropractic, where chiropractic should have considerable control over the training of orthodox doctors. This never happened as the state not only accepted the limitations of the knowledge base of chiropractic, but also denied chiropractic the powers recommended. Statist medicine was then not seriously challenged, even with such opprobrium heaped on the medical profession by the Commissioners.

Chiropractors could be characterised as having an epistemological orientation based on their philosophical conceptions of the development and treatment of disease, and on the use of their practical skills for the public good. Their action orientation, in this instance, was to get access to state-insurance benefits. The Commission accepted the access but without the philosophy. For the medical profession, their epistemological orientation could be characterised as preserving the sanctity of the scientific validation of therapies, and their action orientation was to retain control over the delivery of primary care services. The compromise arrived at by the Commission was the same as with the chiropractors, to reject their epistemological orientation but to accept their action orientation.

Concluding comments

The case of chiropractic provides insight into how therapeutic pluralism is shaped in contemporary Western societies. Chiropractic is well organised and strategically sophisticated in its engagement with its patient population and with the state. In many countries, it has had the ambition to access the same level of state support as the medical profession. It has failed in all cases to achieve this, but it has made substantial gains. In the case of New Zealand, its efforts allowed many chiropractic patients access to state support for their chiropractic treatment.

This chapter demonstrates how difficult it is for an alternative therapy to achieve success in this way. Chiropractic had to give up in its claim to be an alternative system of healing that could act as a primary care profession. Strategically, chiropractic had to walk a fine line between being seen as too radical and being seen as too similar to already established statist healthcare occupations. In effect, we see something like a blunted therapeutic pluralism at this level of therapeutic occupations and organisations. Compromises and accommodations are made, but any real sense of plurality is not achieved.

Similar processes, but sometimes different rhetorical strategies, can be seen in other domains of practice. In a study of how chiropractors are positioned in sports medicine teams in Canada, Nancy Theberge found a tension over their role. These teams could be comprised of a range of therapists, including physicians, physiotherapists, masseurs and chiropractors. Chiropractors could position themselves as primary care practitioners with skills in diagnosis as well as treatment, and resented being categorised as spinal manipulators only. Physicians would be content with chiropractors if they limited their scope of practice and so were 'team players', under the direction of the physician (Theberge 2008). Theberge's study aligns well with the argument made in this chapter, that in order to be accepted and given a legitimated role, chiropractors are required to reduce their scope of practice.

We can also witness a continuity of discursive strategies through to the micro-level of the medical consultation. For example, research shows medical practitioners dissuading patients from going to see their chiropractor for back pain and claiming that chiropractic philosophies of preventive treatment is a fantastic way to make money – a variation on the chiropractors as salesman argument (Dew et al. 2008). This research on consultations took place thirty years after the Commission of Inquiry, highlighting the durability of such critiques.

In both the courts of the United States and in the Commission of Inquiry in New Zealand, statist medicine was found wanting in terms of how it related to chiropractic. Yet in both jurisdictions, chiropractic could only gain limited access to state resources. In the following chapter, the focus shifts from debates and strategies that occur within Western therapeutic systems, to the complex relationship that occurs between competing therapeutic systems when Western and non-Western systems jostle for position in China and when Chinese medicine goes West.

References

Atkinson, P. (1997) *The clinical experience: The construction and reconstruction of clinical reality*, Aldershot: Ashgate.

Baer, H. (2001) *Biomedicine and alternative healing systems in America: Issues of class, race, ethnicity and gender*, Madison: The University of Wisconsin Press.

Baer, H. and Coulter, I. (2008) Taking stock of integrative medicine: Broadening biomedicine or co-option of complementary and alternative medicine?, *Health Sociology Review*, 17, 4, 331–341.

Brosnan, C. (2017) Alternative futures: Fields, boundaries, and divergent professionalisation strategies within the Chiropractic profession, *Social Science & Medicine*, 190, 83–91.

Clavarino, A. and Yates, P. (1995) Fear, faith or rational choice: Understanding the users of alternative therapies, in G. Lupton and J. Najman (eds.), *Sociology of health and illness: Australian readings*, Melbourne: Macmillan, pp. 252–275.

Coburn, D. (1993) State authority, medical dominance, and trends in the regulation of the health professions: The Ontario case, *Social Science & Medicine*, 37, 2, 129–138.

Coburn, D. and Biggs, C.L. (1986) Limits to medical dominance: The case of chiropractic, *Social Science & Medicine*, 22, 10, 1035–1046.

Commission of Inquiry into Chiropractic (1979) *Chiropractic in New Zealand: Report of the commission of inquiry*, Wellington, New Zealand: P. D. Hasselberg, Govt. Printer.

Dew, K. (2000) Apostasy to orthodoxy: Debates before a commission of inquiry into chiropractic, *Sociology of Health and Illness*, 22, 3, 1310–1330.

Dew, K., Plumridge, E., Stubbe, M., Dowell, A., Macdonald, L. and Major, G. (2008) 'You just got to eat healthy': The topic of CAM in the general practice consultation, *Health Sociology Review*, 17, 4, 396–409.

Jamous, H. and Peloille, B. (1970) Changes in the French university-hospital system, in J. Jackson (ed.), *Professions and professionalization*, Cambridge: Cambridge University Press, pp. 111–152.

Potter, J. (1996) *Representing reality: Discourse, rhetoric and social construction*, London: Sage.

Saks, M. (1992) The paradox of incorporation: Acupuncture and the medical profession in modern Britain, in M. Saks (ed.), *Alternative medicine in Britain*, Oxford: Clarendon Press, pp. 183–198.

——— (1994) The alternatives to medicine, in J. Gabe and D. Kelleher (eds.), *Challenging medicine*, London: Routledge, pp. 84–103.

Smith-Cunnien, S.L. (1998) *A profession of one's own: Organized medicine's opposition to chiropractic*, Lanham: University Press of America.

Stinear, J. (1991) Chiropractic: A survivor, *New Zealand Medical Association Newsletter*, 35, 14.

Theberge, N. (2008) The integration of chiropractors into healthcare teams: A case study from sport medicine, *Sociology of Health & Illness*, 30, 1, 19–34.

Turner, B.S. (1987) *Medical power and social knowledge*, London: Sage.

Willis, E. (1983) *Medical dominance: The division of labour in Australian healthcare*, Sydney: George Allen & Unwin.

5

TRANSFORMATION, CONTINUITY AND THE EBB AND FLOW OF CHINESE MEDICINE

The case of Chinese medicine provides a different set of insights into therapeutic pluralism and its possibilities. The developments of Chinese medicine within China and how it has been exported and taken up outside of China demonstrates how one modality can take on different forms and establish different relations between statist medicine and alternative therapeutics. In China, Chinese medicine has at times been part of statist medicine, and at other times, it has had a more tenuous relationship with the state. The export of Chinese medicine to the West has resulted in it being partially incorporated in some states, where it may be supported through education and health benefits. Such incorporation can paradoxically attenuate therapeutic pluralism. The notion of pluralism can be further challenged as an examination of Chinese medicine shows that it is not one entity, it is not singular, and within Chinese medicine there are a plurality of positions, therapeutic activities and representations.

Chinese medicine concepts

It is worth lingering a little on some understandings of the underpinnings of Chinese therapeutics in order to consider its reproduction and transformation over time and in different spaces. By the end of the Han dynasty in AD 220, a system of Chinese medicine was firmly established (Bridgman 1974). Chinese medical concepts are embedded in Confucianism and Taoism. In the oldest Chinese books, the universe is composed of five elements – water, fire, wood, earth and metal – and the universe is a result of a 'great, unchanging, organizing principle' – the Tao (Bridgman 1974: 11). This Tao takes the form of two complementary forces – the yin and the yang. The yin is female, dark, cold and humid, and the yang is male, brilliant, hot and dry. The five elements correspond to the seasons, winds, organs, colours and so forth, and produce each other in a circle of production. Water produces wood which produces fire which produces earth which produces metal. Another energy, qi (or chi or ch'i), permeates everything, and Robert Bridgman argues that in this it is similar to the ether of Western philosophers and physicists (Bridgman 1974). There are twelve channels or meridians, each connected to a main organ. On these meridians are points which are foci of energy and which are influenced by the insertion of needles of various sizes and metals or using moxibustion. In Chinese meridian theory, the channels are unseen but embody a physical reality, and the substances qi and blood move along them (Kaptchuk 1983).

An important element of diagnosis is feeling the pulse (sphygmology), which is characterised quite differently from Western approaches. In particular, taking the pulse at the radial artery is a complex procedure, with many pulses being located on each radial pulse area (as opposed to the one defined in Western medicine), and there are many different qualities associated with each pulse (Chow 1984). Possibly, the first pulses of interest were ones that were called pulses indicative of death (Hsu 2001). Early texts conveyed a sense of the quality of the pulse in figurative ways, such as a pulse that 'seems to bubble under the fingers irregularly like water over a great fire' and a 'pulse seems like a fish, whose head is stopped, and cannot move, but frisks with its tail not very regularly' (Hsu 2001: 195).

Acupuncture is perhaps the most well-known treatment modality used in Chinese medicine known in the West, but it is one amongst many and the major ones are as follows (Chow 1984):

1 Acupuncture – where fine needles are inserted into surface points, of which some 722 are well known. There are theoretical efforts to attribute the clinical success of acupuncture to neurophysiological responses understandable in Western terms, for example, by increasing antibody resistance, affecting the autonomic nervous system or increasing the release of endogenous opiates from the pituitary gland.
2 Acupressure – where the same surface points are treated but with pressure applied from the fingertips.
3 Moxibustion – where moxa sticks, made from rolled leaves of a particular plant, are held over energy points whilst they are burnt.
4 Remedial massage – a pressing and rubbing massage (An-Mo) and a thrusting and rolling massage (Tui-na) to produce effects at organs and upon organ function.
5 Cupping – where heated jars are applied to body points in order to disperse congestion.
6 Respiratory exercise – to regulate the circulation of the blood and the breath.
7 Physical exercise – where external and internal balance is maintained while in movement (Tai Chi).
8 Herb medicine – where Chinese herbs are used to treat conditions. The number of medical formulas identified in Chinese medicine number nearly 100,000, but in practice Chinese physicians may use just a handful of these (Scheid 2002).

Arguably, an important contrast between Chinese medicine and biomedicine is in the role that the patient plays. Judith Farquhar (1994: 45) argues that in Chinese medicine 'the doctor does not have the power to reject any sign reported by the patient' and so patients retain an authority not so obviously held in Western medicine.

Another contrast is the way in which bodily structures can be given an agency in Chinese medicine that does not have any equivalence in biomedicine. The liver, for example, is described as being 'responsible' for the sinews, being responsible for fright, and of making strategies (Scheid 2002: 50). The liver then is envisaged as a conscious agent not just an organ that reacts in physiologically determined ways.

Paul Unschuld (1992) suggests that understandings of knowledge production and truth are grounded in quite different ways in the West and in China. Whereas in the West there is a notion of one truth, and that scientific development can mean the overturning of old ways of seeing the world for a new one, as in Kuhnian scientific revolutions, in China the grounding was more in a firm establishment of truth, from the Han dynasty, with further developments and growth in knowledge building on that base. From this perspective, the process of taking in Western science into a Chinese perspective would seem a likely outcome of the confrontation between Western medicine and TCM, rather than one displacing the other.

From a Western medical perspective, Chinese medicine suffered from two major weaknesses (Bridgman 1974). One is that there was no development of the study of anatomy. In China, there existed Confucian religious and ethical prohibitions against dissection (Kaptchuk 1983). A second weakness is that surgery was barred due to an edict forbidding the mutilation of the body. According to Chinese thought, 'your physical being was a gift from your parents and to harm or disfigure it in any way was viewed as a grossly unfilial act' (Cohen 1974: 78)

In the Chinese sciences motion and change are taken as given and therefore do not need to be explained but, on the other hand, stasis and fixity do need explanation.

> Chinese medicine heals in a world of unceasing transformation. This condition of constant change, this fluidity of material forms, stands in sharp contrast to a (modern Western) commonsense world of discrete entities characterized by fixed essences, which seem to be exhaustively describable in structural terms.
>
> *(Farquhar 1994: 24)*

For the expert practitioner, Chinese medicine is a virtuoso practice combining the 'authenticity' of ancient medical texts with the specifics of the case, making for a dynamic process that is not formulaic (Farquhar 1992).

A distinctive aspect of Chinese medicine diagnosis is pattern recognition and differentiation. Pattern differentiation is not the same as disease recognition. Some diseases can express themselves through different patterns, and some diseases might require different treatments according to the pattern prescribed (Scheid 2002). Pattern recognition was not systemised until the 1950s, in response to events outlined in the following section.

Chinese medicine at home

Chinese government initiatives have fostered some level of incorporation of Chinese medicine into the medical school curricula, the availability of it in hospitals and other healthcare settings and the modernising of the processing and packaging of TCM remedies (Quah 2008).

However, acupuncture and TCM have had a variable history, even in their place of origin. Cullen (1993) argues that in the sixteenth century acupuncture and moxibustion were not the therapies used by the literate healers of China but were used by lower status people with little medical learning. Rather, the literate healers prescribed drugs, of which the patients expected a rapid cure. Cullen also claims that remedies were given to deal with external pathogenic agents. Chinese therapeutics in the sixteenth century seems surprisingly modern, with the exception that if a healer failed to cure in one or two attempts, another healer, perhaps of a different persuasion, would be called in. Perhaps that is not so different to what we have today, as I will consider in Chapter 7. Even prior to Western incursions into China aspects of TCM could be despised, for example, in 1822 an imperial edict prohibited the Imperial Medical Academy from teaching or practicing acupuncture (Barnes 2005)

Efforts to legitimate Chinese medicine in China took different forms. One was to suggest that what was useful in TCM and Western medicine could be adapted in therapeutic approaches. Another was arguments made that the original Chinese texts, before misinterpretation over the centuries, contained approaches that aligned with Western medicine. Another approach was to align TCM with dialectical materialism. The purchase of these arguments waxed and waned over time.

In the early twentieth century, Western medical ideas started to make a major impact on the medical system in China, at first through public health concepts. Carl Nathan argues that the North Manchurian Plague Prevention Service was China's first regional medical programme 'run according to principles called "modern" in the West' (Nathan 1974: 56). In 1910, the pneumonic plague spread terror in Manchuria and took a toll of 60,000 lives. Claims were made that there was a fifty percent mortality rate among practitioners of Chinese medicine and only two percent among practitioners of Western medicine (Sidel 1983). The plague developed particularly amongst marmot trappers, who flooded into Manchuria to trap this rodent for Western markets. The marmots were plague infested. Once caught, the pneumonic plague is transmitted directly between people (as opposed to the bubonic plague which requires fleas) and in 1910 there was no remedy. The only intervention was to 'segregate the dying from the healthy' (Nathan 1974: 57). As Chinese medicine seemed powerless against this terrifying outbreak of the disease, authorities from the emperor on down resorted to modern preventive measures, a move that was unpopular as it appeared to give superiority to modern Western medicine.

The importance of the wider political context in the establishment of relations between the medical professions and the state is evident from this. In addition, public health measures only became a necessity as a consequence of the development of rail links leading to the Manchurian frontier which meant the plague could spread (Cohen 1974). One form of modernisation necessitated the importation of other forms, so giving a foothold for Western medicine in China.

The impact of Western medicine manifested in its uptake by state institutions in China. For the first half of the twentieth century Chinese medicine was under hostile attack in China. The link between modernisation and medicine was made even more explicit by the activities of the Rockefeller Foundation who developed medical programmes in China. Proponents of a China programme argued that 'Western medicine was the vehicle by which to move China from a medieval condition to a modern nation' (Bowers 1974: 85). The Rockefeller Foundation established the China Medical Board in 1914, with its main priority being the development of the Peking Union Medical College. Simon Flexner, the brother of Abraham Flexner who was responsible for the Flexner Report in the United States, noted in Chapter 2, was the director of the Rockefeller Institute and was involved in the Second China Medical Commission in 1915. This commission recommended linking up the best Western medical schools with research programmes in China (Bowers 1974: 87). English was recommended as the language of instruction. A medical elite was established that was not created to serve the needs of the population at large in China and was restricted to instruction in a foreign language, so undermining the native culture and the native medical traditions. Peking Union Medical College personnel dominated the Chinese Medical Association and the Chinese Academy of Medical Sciences, the latter being the centralised organ for medical research. Graduates became presidents and vice-presidents of many other medical colleges in China (Brown Bullock 1974).

By 1922, traditionalists were ranked lower than modernists by the Ministry of the Interior, and seven years later, the Ministry of Health resolved to abolish the old medicine entirely (Nathan 1974). Unschuld argues that a powerful reason for the embracing of Western medicine in China and the downgrading of TCM followed a series of major defeats to Western powers. Western science was regarded as a solution to regaining the strength of the nation (Unschuld 1992). Efforts by Western medicine physicians failed to outlaw it in 1929, but many colleges of Chinese medicine were closed. Chinese medicine had lost political power, but was still popular in everyday life (Scheid 2002). This negative view of Chinese medicine led to the traditionalists lobbying, and by 1935, the National government resolved to accord equal status to Chinese and Western style doctors.

In the 1950s, there was a rapid influx from the Soviet Union of 'consultants, technology, and methods of organization' remoulding the Chinese system of medicine into a Soviet style system (Sidel 1974: 106). Prior to Mao Zedong coming to power in 1949, most physicians in China were trained as apprentices in TCM (Weiss and Lonnquist 2012). In 1949, Chairman Mao called for the amalgamation of the two streams of medicine (traditional Chinese and Western) under 'one universal physical system' (Chow 1984: 120). Chinese medicine then transformed into a therapeutic approach taught and practiced through state-controlled institutions, replacing the apprenticeship training or private school training that had prevailed before, and its practice in private clinics and hospitals (Scheid 2002). Support from Mao Zedong for Chinese medicine is thought to derive in part from his own personal experience of it during the Long March of 1935. Chinese medicine was used to successfully treat Mao's inflamed joints after Western medicine had failed to offer respite (Scheid 2002).

After 1949, several initiatives were introduced to respond to a lack of health resources, particularly in rural areas. One initiative was to foster the use of Western medicine alongside Chinese medicine. In 1958, China introduced a system of chìjiǎo yīshēng, or barefoot doctors, which was a system of rural health workers who undertook a range of activities, including anti-epidemic work. The training of barefoot doctors took substantially less time than the training of conventional doctors and could be part-time and on-the-job (Koplan et al. 1985). They were trained in both Western medicine and traditional Chinese approaches (Lee 1997). Healthcare personnel were trained at an astonishing rate, as opposed to the elitist training at the Peking Union Medical College, and there was a rapid increase in the number of hospitals (Sidel 1974). Despite these efforts, the Ministry of Health was still identified as being urban, elitist, anti-TCM and following foreign forms of education. Mao, in 1965, claimed that the Ministry of Health 'should be called the Urban Public Health Ministry of the Privileged' (Sidel 1974: 111).

It was in the 1950s that the term traditional Chinese medicine (TCM) was first used in Chinese publications, but it was used for foreign language publications. The term traditional Chinese medicine, abbreviated to TCM, was coined by the People's Republic of China in an effort to globally promote this therapeutic approach (Leung 2008). Whereas within China there was an emphasis on the new, so putting 'traditional' in front of Chinese Medicine would have given it a derogatory connotation, for Westerners continuity with a venerable past was to be emphasised (Scheid 2002). Unschuld claims that TCM was never a coherent system unchanged through history, and that contemporary commenters on TCM neglect aspects that be found in TCM writings, such as demonological and religious aspects (Unschuld 1992). Geomancy is a less well-known aspect of Chinese medicine. The health of descendants is connected to the health of ancestors, and so there is a need to ensure the propitious burial of ancestors and geomancy is used to achieve this. In China today, geomancers may identify the proper sites for burial and the proper orientation of the grave, based on cosmological understandings and ideas of correspondence between the human body and the structures of the earth (Seaman 1992). Such aspects of Chinese medicine are not so evident in the Western world's reception of TCM.

The idea of a single new medicine, rather than cooperation between Chinese and Western medicine, was a goal until around 1956, but during this period the Western influenced Ministry of Health ensured that Chinese medicine maintained its inferior status. Chinese medicine was viewed by these modernisers as the medicine of a feudal society. Chinese medical practitioners were required to be licensed from 1952 and had to pass state-controlled exams that required knowledge of Western medicine. Chinese medicine Improvement Schools were established that had as one of their goals raising levels of knowledge of Western medicine (Scheid 2002). This negative view of Chinese medicine was overturned in 1953 with policies to expand the scope of Chinese medicine that included incorporating it into hospitals and national insurance schemes. Volker Scheid (2002) argues that this reversal can be linked to a number of shifts in sentiment, including a sense of national pride and a desire to be less dependent on imported technology. Under Mao Zedong's edicts physicians practicing Western medicine were now to learn Chinese medicine through re-education classes initiated in 1955. The goal was to establish a medicine that would be a new medicine for the world (Scheid 2002).

However, in the process of modernisation new textbooks on Chinese medicine were created, that rendered the traditional form of Chinese medicine education of studying the classic texts void. More serious consequences for Chinese medicine occurred with the cultural revolution of 1966–1976. Formal education was under siege and ceased in Chinese medical colleges, and the Western medical sector came more into favour. The classical roots of Chinese medicine were despised, and classical texts were burned in bonfires (Scheid 2002).

After 1976 and the end of the cultural revolution, there was yet another shift. Socialism was to be established with a Chinese character, providing new possibilities for Chinese classical culture, and a plural healthcare system was to be developed (Scheid 2002). By the 1980s, the official position was now that Chinese medicine, Western medicine and integrated Chinese and Western medicine should co-exist and be supported (Scheid 2002). However, although Chinese medicine and Western medicine schools both had state support, the latter were regarded as more prestigious and were more difficult to get into (Scheid 2002). And although Chinese medicine hospitals are state supported, they make up only a small percentage of total hospitals (Scheid 2002).

The socialist principles underlying the delivery of Chinese health care up to the 1980s meant that efforts were made to provide health care free or at low cost with most funding coming from the government. This changed in the 1980s with a shift towards a market-oriented economy, which has placed much healthcare delivery into private ownership, and where most of the funding comes from fees for service charges to patients or health insurance companies (Weiss and Lonnquist 2012). The barefoot doctor system no longer operated. However, trading in traditional Chinese medications flourished, with medical retailers and distributors outnumbering practitioners (Ooi 1991).

How Chinese medicine is positioned at a discursive level can also operate to limit its clinical use and disempower it in the state-supported health system.

Physicians in Chinese hospitals would be reluctant to treat life-threatening conditions with Chinese medicine alone, even if they believed it might be the best option, because if the patient died they would face accusations of neglect for not using Western medicine, accusations that would not be defended by any authority. The same would not apply if physicians used Western medicine alone and the patient died (Scheid 2002).

The term 'orchestrated medical pluralism' has been used to capture the relationship between therapeutic practices in China (Scheid 2002). Orchestrated medical pluralism can be viewed as a process of Chinese medicine, in this instance, accommodating to state demands of standardising practices and aligning with the assumptions of scientific medicine in order to survive (Scheid 2002). The state demands simplifications and standardisation in the implementation of education and research, in order to justify the spending of resources on Chinese medicine. That is, Chinese medicine must make these accommodations to become embedded in what I have been referring to as statist medicine. These processes can be understood within a broader understanding of the state as articulated by theorists such as Theodore Porter (1995) and John Scott (1998). Over many centuries, there have been developments that render intelligible and legible social practices, like the standardising of weights and measures to facilitate the legibility of the exchange of goods and services. This process of increasing legibility allows for greater oversight by organisations and institutions, such as the state, that may be distant from where such social practices occur. Similarly, processes of simplification and standardisation render the therapeutic practices of individuals more legible to the state (Dew 2012). Some of the detail of these processes are clearly outlined by Scheid (2002), such as the Chinese Ministry of Health promoting the standardisation of disease classification in Chinese medicine, and publications and organisations promoting Chinese medicine being overseen by the state through the Ministry of Health.

In the post-Maoist era, an emphasis on science and technology further promoted this process of standardisation of Chinese medicine. By 1995, national standards for the approach taken to 406 different diseases were adopted in teaching and research institutions. Other standardising processes continued, including the standardising of clinical terminology in 1997. In doing so, the state could administer disease records and undertake statistical analyses (Scheid 2002). The state now could 'see' and better control Chinese medicine. However, this seeing has its limitations as physicians claim an artistry in linking disease mechanisms, pattern descriptions, diagnosis and prescription (Scheid 2002).

There are other forces of change and continuity, in addition to political forces and standardisation processes. Scheid (2002) suggests that for all observers, including Western social scientists, Chinese politicians, practitioners and patients, Chinese medicine is categorically different now compared to what it was in the imperial era. Simple technological changes to the production of stainless steel needles for acupuncture means that needling practices have changed, with deeper needling more readily used, and electronic needle stimulators changing the interaction between the patient and the physician (Scheid 2002). But needling remains a skill that has to be acquired over years of practice, and so an example of an aspect of practice that is not so easily standardised. The limits of standardisation are also revealed in the undisciplined and creative practices of practitioners.

Over the twentieth century, there was a shift from an apprenticeship system as the form of instruction to college instruction, but Scheid (2002) notes that this distinction is not absolute as Chinese medicine students are placed in internships with an established physician, and therefore the importance of personal transmission and practice is still retained. The master-pupil relationship is based on the filial relationship between father and son, a relationship that has responsibilities and obligation quite different from a Western teacher-student relationship.

There are different understandings of what this kind of relationship might imply. Concerns are raised that the master-disciple relationship is one of the imitations where students are turned into copies of their masters and where there is an aversion to critical inquiry. A contrasting view is that the practice of Chinese medicine is an art, where the student can come to learn and understand that which cannot be captured in words (Scheid 2002). That is, there are tensions here between standardisation processes and that which evades standardising procedures and techniques.

The use of Chinese medicine in Chinese hospitals remains quite diverse and non-standardised, despite state efforts. Scheid suggests that ten Chinese medicine physicians would suggest ten different prescriptions for the same condition (Scheid 2002). This variability is not seen as a problem, but the diversity is welcomed. In Chinese universities, there are at least seven different methods of pattern variation taught, pattern variation being seen by many as a distinctive foundation of Chinese medicine (Scheid 2002). This form of diagnosis is in addition to biomedical diagnostic teaching. Differences of opinion abound about the meaning of diagnostic findings, such as the link between pulses and visceral systems.

In domestic spaces in Chinese households, Chinese medicine can be an everyday practice. Big Leung talks of being brought up in a household where herbal teas and soups were often used with the goal of promoting health, and in cities with a predominantly Chinese population many shops sold herbal drinks and Chinese remedies (Leung 2008) Chinese migrants in Australia and elsewhere would adjust their everyday habits to keep in balance with their environment, for example, eating yang foods in winter and yin foods in summer. Adolescent girls were given yin soups to prepare them for pregnancy and breast feeding, or TCM for nourishing yin. Soups, based on TCM principles, were commonly used for therapeutic purposes, with one women stating that in her family 'I was always having soups for this and soups for that' (Leung 2008: 122), with this knowledge of food and soups passed down through the generations. Within these immigrant communities, there were also folk or subaltern aspects to their relationship to TCM. Knowledge about remedies and approaches could be passed down through families or through apprenticeships, and in some cases, this knowledge was jealously guarded (Leung 2008). And taking care of oneself was a filial duty, as bodies were 'gifts from their parents' (Leung 2008: 137).

In research on Chinese migrants in Australia, it was found that they use TCM and biomedicine in a complementary way. For some participants in the research, biomedicine was used for acute situations, and for surgery, and TCM was used in a preventive way, to strengthen the body and nourish energy, or for chronic conditions, and was viewed as having fewer side effects (Leung 2008). Biomedicine could be used for conditions that were described in the terms of TCM, such as using biomedicine for 'pain due to wind' and TCM was seen as more appropriate for 'pain in bones' (Leung 2008: 37). Biomedicine was seen as a problem-specific approach whereas TCM was a whole person approach.

The standard story about the use of Western medicine and Chinese medicine is that the former is best for acute conditions, such as infectious diseases and situations requiring surgery, whereas the latter is better for chronic conditions and as a preventive. However, Scheid observes that patient practices in China belie such simple dichotomies. Rather than people holding different beliefs about what conditions are best suited to what therapeutic modality decisions about whether to go to a Western physician or a Chinese physician can result from complex interacting concerns. These concerns may include what other family members believe, past experiences, preferences for pills or decoctions, willingness to prepare medication or not and so on (Scheid 2002). But even within China, there are regional differences in the popular receptivity of Chinese medicine, and where Chinese medicine is a component of everyday cooking it is more openly received (Scheid 2002). There are understandings that bodies are different in different environments. In southern China, people are less receptive of harsh Chinese medications than those in the north as they believe that their constitutions are more delicate resulting from, at least in part, climatic difference (Scheid 2002).

In sum, in China, there has been a complex process of state support and state suppression, and of change to Chinese medicine as well as continuity, but also the retention of distinct epistemologies, ontologies and forms of therapeutic instruction. Although organised therapeutic pluralism captures some of this, especially the link between state recognition and standardisation, there is still something undisciplined in the artistry of Chinese therapeutic practices and in the incorporation of therapeutic understandings into everyday life.

Chinese medicine goes West

The recorded presence of Chinese therapeutic practices in the West goes back hundreds of years. In the thirteenth century, William Rubruck, a friar dispatched to China by Louis IX of France, noted that Chinese physicians knew a great deal about herbs and could diagnose very cleverly from the pulse. In 1683, the first medical essay on acupuncture written for the West appeared (Barnes 2005). In

Europe, in the eighteenth century, particularly in France, there was a positive reception given to moxibustion in the treatment of gout. This was in part due to the differences between the systems of medicine being rather narrower at that time than they were later, and the capacity to translate the effects of moxibustion into Western understandings, such as being akin to cautery. Acupuncture however did not gain much purchase as the idea of puncturing the skin had no analogous mechanisms in Western medicine at that time (Bivins 2007). By the nineteenth century, acupuncture gained wider acceptance in Europe, in part due to the observable success in treating ailments like muscular pain and nervous conditions, ailments that had a prominent place in the medical marketplace at the time (Bivins 2007). The clinical success of the treatment overrode any possible concerns about explanations for its action. The spread of acupuncture in France and England was fostered by socially prominent individuals who had experienced relief from symptoms by the treatment and medical practitioners who wanted to add the technique to their armoury. However, its time in the limelight was brief as the reporting of single cases in the medical press, which had stimulated interest in acupuncture, went out of fashion (Bivins 2007). Single case narratives are used in medical instruction to provide insights into reasoning styles (Scheid 2002), something that has less status in the Western scientific method.

Unlike homeopathy during the nineteenth century in England, there were no centres of training established that was based on acupuncture. Today, the education and regulation of Chinese medicine and acupuncture vary greatly throughout the world. In the Australian state of Victoria, an occupational licensing scheme for TCM practitioners was introduced in 2000 (Possamai-Inesedy and Cochrane 2013). Licensing laws can have unanticipated consequences, with licensed practitioners being the only therapists allowed to practice acupuncture. Other therapists, such as physiotherapists and massage therapists, use 'dry needling' instead, thus avoiding being censured for using acupuncture (Possamai-Inesedy and Cochrane 2013). Dry needling looks like acupuncture but is based on the idea of stimulating trigger points and not influencing qi. Regulation of Chinese herbs can also have paradoxical consequences. In Australia, the Therapeutic Goods Authority assessed some Chinese herbs as toxic. In doing so, the herbs become inaccessible to the expert Chinese herbalists who use them in their traditional healing context but are available to medical doctors with lower levels of training and who can use them in ways divorced from traditional understandings (Possamai-Inesedy and Cochrane 2013).

In the early 1970s, public interest was generated in America by acupuncture. American medical teams went to China to study acupuncture and brought back reports of its success, particularly in anaesthesia. Due to this publicity, acupuncture in America became popular, drawing resources away from the orthodox practitioners (Berliner 1984). This situation was remedied in most states by the passing of legislation that required non-physician acupuncturists to work under the supervision of licensed doctors (Freund and McGuire 1991), though the passing of this legislation was accomplished in large part due to the efforts of acupuncture organisations and clientele (Chow 1984). In addition to licensing and training of Chinese medicine practitioners, many orthodox medical practitioners picked up Chinese medical practices and by the mid-1980s about 3,000 American medical doctors were involved in acupuncture (Baer 2001). Thus, acupuncture, even with its conflicting epistemology, was co-opted by scientific medicine in the United States. However, there are acupuncturists who operate outside of the licensing system, the subaltern practitioners who ply their trade in such places as the backrooms of gift shops in Chinatowns in US cities (Baer 2001).

In France, medically trained doctors who have achieved acupuncture accreditation can practice acupuncture and it is illegal for others to do so, an approach followed by Portugal with approval for medical doctors being achieved in 2002, whereas prior to that there was no legal protection for the practice of acupuncture (Almeida 2012).

Whatever the different regulatory arrangement around acupuncture and TCM, its impact on the non-Chinese societies is evident. There are many Western universities offering degrees in Chinese medicine, there is a hospital in Germany staffed by physicians from a Chinese Medicine hospital in Beijing and tens of thousands of foreign students are taught Chinese medicine in Chinese universities (Scheid 2002).

Ted Kaptchuk (1983: 1) tells a story told in China, where a maintenance man who had worked in a Western missionary hospital returned to his village to set himself up as a health practitioner using Western therapeutics, that is, hypodermic needles and antibiotics. Many people got well despite his lack of knowledge of Western therapeutics. Kaptchuk argues that something similar happens in the West, where some basic techniques of TCM are used and people get well, '[b] ut the theoretical depth and full clinical potential of Chinese medicine remain virtually unknown'.

This view is tempered by research from several Western countries, which provides a slightly more nuanced picture. Research in Norway found that many medical practitioners who used acupuncture used TCM concepts in understanding their practice rather than using standard scientific explanations (Sagli 2001). For many, these concepts referred to a reality that was then different from a biomedical one, with concepts like qi (energy or vital force), jingluo (meridians) and zangfu (bodily networks) being used (Sagli 2001). Kaptchuk's concern about a lack of theoretical depth may of course still apply but this research does suggest that practitioners are integrating or assimilating some aspects of TCM.

In a study of German medical doctors who used acupuncture, it was found that there was a variety of approaches to its use (Frank and Stollberg 2004). A minority of these medical acupuncturists used acupuncture in selected cases, particularly in cases of chronic pain which was a condition covered by health insurance companies. Some used acupuncture, biomedicine and a range of other modalities. Rarely, medical acupuncturists explained needling in biomedical terms, such as acupuncture stimulating the release of endogenous opiates. More commonly, medical acupuncturists described biomedicine's effects and other alternative practices' effects using Chinese concepts – such as the five elements, meridians and qi. The choice of which particular therapy to use could be quite pragmatic, for example, moxibustion would be avoided by some because of its smell, and herbal remedies based on Chinese pharmacology might be little used because of the difficulty in accessing the herbs (Frank and Stollberg 2004).

Chinese medicine then has variable uptake in different countries and occupies different positions in relation to the state, with acupuncture being a major focus for many medical practitioners. We now turn to an exploration of the kind of discursive work that medical acupuncturists undertook to become securely embedded in the medical profession.

Deviant insiders and medical acupuncture

Acupuncture is now a widely used form of treatment, and there are many medical doctors who specialise in acupuncture. The incorporation of acupuncture into medical practice continues to be disputed. Supporters of medical acupuncture can suggest that if medical practitioners are not around who can use it then patients will attend lay practitioners who do not have the same grounding in differential diagnosis and cannot use the array of therapeutic options open to a medical practitioner. Those who oppose its use in established medicine can be concerned that if you let medical practitioners use acupuncture, where will it end? The boundaries of acceptable practice might start to be redrawn, a similar issue to allowing chiropractors access to state support.

This section looks at the arguments made in orthodox medical journals about medical acupuncture and compares those with the ways in which medical acupuncturists discuss their therapy amongst themselves, in their own journals and newsletters. The material is primarily taken from New Zealand medical journals and associated publications during a time when medical acupuncturists were attempting to become incorporated into the New Zealand Medical Association (Dew 2000). This comparison is very informative as it gives us a chance to see the way in which acupuncture can be presented quite differently and the kind of work that these different presentations do. The way in which acupuncture is described is as much political as it is philosophical or practical. These comparisons also demonstrate that the medical profession does not speak with one voice or take one stance on issues relating to alternative medicine, and that there is not as much unity within the medical profession as might be thought. I am focusing here on the representations of acupuncture in text and considering the work that such textual or discursive representations perform.

As noted, in the West acupuncture in particular gained much public attention in the early 1970s after a number of Western orthodox physicians returned from China with eye-witness accounts of its marvels (Berliner 1984). The sudden interest in acupuncture in the West caught the medical profession off guard (Wolpe 1985). There were debates over whether acupuncture should be placed in the hands of orthodox medical practitioners who could label themselves medical acupuncturists, or whether it should be excluded from medicine completely. Prior to these reports in the 1970s, medical journals in English-speaking countries questioned reports of the efficacy of acupuncture. It was of particular concern that the concepts used in TCM, such as qi and the meridians, had no counterpart in Western neurological and physiological models.

Medical physicians who witnessed acupuncture treatments in China argued that scientific evaluation of acupuncture should be undertaken. In 1974, members of a New Zealand medical delegation sent to China were impressed with acupuncture anaesthesia but were unimpressed with acupuncture diagnosis and with moxibustion. Others in the medical profession used editorials, opinion pieces and letters to the editor in medical journals to express their disdain of acupuncture, drawing on standard critiques of CAM therapeutics such as that any therapeutic success of acupuncture must be a result of the placebo effect and that acupuncture was one of many pseudoscience practices. Cultural and political concerns were also apparent, seen in the claim that acupuncture was a cultural technique aimed at establishing and advancing Chinese cultural values.

The fear that lay acupuncturists would monopolise acupuncture was expressed. The term lay practitioner is used here to describe someone who practises acupuncture or TCM but who has not got a medical degree. This does not mean they are untrained, but they are not trained as medical doctors first. It was claimed that the techniques of lay practitioners should be studied by the medical profession, so that it would not become 'the prerogative of those unable to make an adequate differential diagnosis' (Gluckman 1973: 325). The diagnostic validity of Western medicine is assumed as the only possible form of diagnosis. This concern about lay practitioners supposed inability to diagnose was used by medical acupuncturists to push for recognition of their own associations within the medical profession.

Medical acupuncturists rhetorically worked to reinforce medical orthodoxy and assuage the concerns of their medical colleagues. A president of a medical acupuncture society claimed that 'most of the old acupuncture points and theories correlate with our modern knowledge of physiology, pathology, anatomy and embryology' (Tseung 1975: 278). At the first conference of the Medical Acupuncture Society, the president emphasised that acupuncture 'did not present any rivalry to established medical practice, and acupuncture could never reverse any pathology, the principles of conventional medicine and surgery remained all-important in total patient management' (New Zealand Medical Journal 1982: 394). In a similar vein to chiropractic, medical acupuncture had presented a de-radicalised face to the medical profession and made claims of a limited applicability of the therapy. In order to be seen as acceptable, acupuncture also had to pose no threat to conventional medical practice.

Claims and counterclaims about the efficacy of acupuncture continued for many years in the *New Zealand Medical Journal*, following a number of themes. A major theme was one of effectiveness. Those who supported acupuncture argued that the evaluation of acupuncture by scientific trials showed its effectiveness for some conditions. A corollary of this argument was that acupuncture was limited in its application, and therefore did not threaten the medical profession's monopoly on the treatment of organic diseases.

The notion of the placebo was an important element in this argument about effectiveness. Opponents of acupuncture argued that studies had not separated out placebo effects and passage of time effects from acupuncture treatment. Allied to this were criticisms of the design of any studies carried out to investigate acupuncture. A claim was made that experiments which indicated that acupuncture led to the release of neurotransmitters proved nothing as 'a well aimed kick on the posterior' may do the same (Malloch 1984: 201). One argued that 'true double-blind acupuncture trials are impossible, as are trials involving a blind operator' (Dowson 1985: 29). Supporters of acupuncture argued that this critique made of acupuncture could also have been levelled at pharmacological agents, surgery and many other treatments commonly used in orthodox medicine.

These arguments were frequently in response to medical research that gave support or questioned the effectiveness of acupuncture, for example, in anaesthesia, post-operative care and for the treatment of migraines. When the researchers concluded that acupuncture had an effect, medical practitioners who opposed acupuncture claimed that there were weaknesses in the research design that invalidated the findings. Conversely, when researchers concluded that acupuncture showed no effect supporters of medical acupuncture would claim that the research design biased the results. No experiment was accepted by all as confirming or denying the usefulness of acupuncture.

Opponents argued that acupuncture is pseudo-scientific rubbish and if it gained acceptance the profession could not keep out other pseudo-scientific practices such as colour therapy, radioasthesia, chiropractic, homoeopathy and witchcraft. This is a thin-end-of-the-wedge argument, where the concern is to stop other therapies taking the same route to acceptability if recognition is conferred upon acupuncture. Others argued that there were other orthodox techniques that were a more conveniently applied equivalent of acupuncture, such as trans-cutaneous neural stimulation. The implication was that these orthodox techniques were scientific, whereas acupuncture was not. Such a view completely eschews the possibility of different ontological understandings, translating acupuncture to some form of nerve stimulation.

The market position of acupuncture was another theme. Opponents argued that acupuncture's attraction was the lure of the easy dollar and it deceived both the doctor and the patient. In addition, taxpayer money should not be wasted on acupuncture (Dew 2000). These themes echo the critiques of chiropractic made by statist medicine noted in Chapter 4.

From these debates, it can be argued that in order to avoid a charge of being a deviant practitioner, medical acupuncturists portrayed themselves as adopting acupuncture techniques, but of rejecting the philosophy of TCM. Acupuncture was reduced from a therapy with general applications, to a therapy with very specific applications in areas where orthodox medicine had not been very successful anyway. Any hint of a threat to those who had years of orthodox medical training had to be removed, and a place was sought within the profession. The medical profession could derive benefit from giving some acceptance to medical acupuncturists. It meant that doctors could refer patients to acupuncture within their own profession, thus controlling it. Although the debate was often about the scientific basis of acupuncture, this can be seen in the case of acupuncture as a rhetorical device employed by those on both sides of the argument. That is, both sides argued that science was on their side. Science was something invoked to support the arguments made, but science was not something that could definitively validate or invalidate the therapy.

Despite the arguments against it, the New Zealand Medical Acupuncture Society was incorporated into the New Zealand Medical Association in 1981, conferring some medical legitimacy to the technique. The way in which medical acupuncture was accommodated by the medical profession in New Zealand has similarities to developments in other countries such as the United Kingdom (Saks 1995) and the United States (Wolpe 1985). However, this public presentation of medical acupuncture as a limited therapeutic tool that could be explained in orthodox medical terms belied the intense debate that was occurring within medical acupuncture circles, to which I will now turn.

Medical acupuncturists talk amongst themselves

Whereas debates in medical journals give an impression of medical acupuncturists using acupuncture in ways which were not too distant from the philosophies of orthodox medicine, the medical acupuncture journals and newsletters show that many medical acupuncturists were far from orthodox. When medical acupuncturists have other medical acupuncturists as an audience, as opposed to the audience being their orthodox medical colleagues, the narrative changes. We can identify several different debates in this context.

As opposed to re-framing Chinese medicine's concepts in physiologically orthodox ways, some medical acupuncturists articulated a concern about needing a deeper understanding of TCM. It was suggested that medical acupuncturists needed to develop a core of traditionally trained acupuncturists in order to prevent criticism from lay acupuncturists that they do not have a good understanding of Chinese medicine (Steeper 1985: 2). Related to the concern about a shallow learning base was a concern that some medical acupuncturists thought that all that was needed to master acupuncture was a short course. Alternative positions to this concern were offered, such as arguments for the superiority of medical acupuncture. Lay acupuncturists, from this perspective, did not have the sound medical knowledge that allowed medical doctors to acquire acupuncture skills more quickly.

Medical acupuncturist talking amongst themselves articulated a more critical approach to the evidence hierarchy in medicine. A host of potential problems with clinical trials that may 'rig' the outcome was noted. These included that in clinical trials for acupuncture the patients selected had usually failed to respond to conventional drug or physical therapy. They were then the most difficult cases to treat and so would be less likely to be responsive to acupuncture. Additionally, few studies used qualified traditional acupuncturists to treat in the way they would in clinical practice, and commonly the treatment provided was formulaic and the number of treatments restricted. This also meant that there was no allowance made to adjust treatment in response to the specific requirements of the patient's condition. Comparisons were also difficult as there were problems finding a suitable placebo, and the ideal of a double-blind trial was not possible as the practitioner could not be ignorant about whether they were delivering the treatment or a placebo. The problem highlighted is that trials take an approach where a formula is developed for treatments of specific conditions, but central to TCM is an approach where specific treatments are developed for each individual patient.

These diverse viewpoints from those in different social locations in the healthcare system reinforce that acupuncture is not a single phenomenon, but that there are a variety of acupunctures. Some medical acupuncturists claimed it worked through known physiological mechanisms and others that concepts like qi could not be translated into orthodox neurological or physiological concepts. Yet others saw developments in the use of acupuncture in the West, such as Electroacupuncture by Voll, a method developed by a German medical doctor in the 1950s that allegedly measured the electrical resistance of acupuncture points, as methods to question the subconscious mind. An editor of the *New Zealand Journal of Acupuncture* provided yet another take on the practice of acupuncture, arguing that for the experienced acupuncturist it can be the 'intention' of the application that is 'just as important as where the needle is placed' and that 'when one needles a person, one not only introduces the needle, but also some of one's own energy as well' (Wong 1991: 2). Perspectives like this can be found in Chinese medicine in China today that is based on centuries old understandings that some kind of spirit connects the physician's hand to their heart when inserting needles (Scheid 2002).

Given the diversity of medical acupuncture, it was not always easy to maintain a coherent stance on issues. For example, in 1986, the inaugural meeting of the World Federation of Acupuncture took place. At this first meeting, the Federation took the position that lay acupuncturists could be included under its constitution. This stance was taken to accommodate the important place that lay acupuncturists had in health systems in some countries, most notably in China and Japan. However, as a result of this decision some medical acupuncture societies in Europe and the Australian society refused to join the Federation. For some medical acupuncturists and societies, if lay acupuncturists could be so easily affiliated to the World Federation and have the same rights as the medical acupuncturists then the World Federation's standards were too low (Dew 2003).

As with chiropractors, discussed in Chapter 4, medical acupuncturists had to balance between opposing forces. Were they to be scientific, traditional or psychodynamic? Were they superior or inferior to lay practitioners? One important plank in their efforts to gain recognition was to set themselves up as the first line of defence against possible incursions from lay practitioners.

The case of medical acupuncture gives an insight into the different sets of problems that arise for the deviant insiders, those who are medically trained but embrace a CAM modality, and the different strategies employed to remain on the inside. One could de-radicalise acupuncture, and turn it into an orthodox form of therapy, or one could embrace deviance, but at the risk of a great cost. Michael Saks (1995: 220) notes that in Britain medical acupuncture had narrowed its scope of application during the 1970s and increasingly subscribed to an orthodox neurophysiological account of acupuncture. New Zealand medical acupuncturists represented acupuncture in this narrowed way during efforts to affiliate with the New Zealand Medical Association. If the orthodox face of acupuncture was what was being promoted, it was safer to have it inside the profession rather than to risk lay practitioners making inroads into the medical profession's territory.

In contrast to the chiropractors, the medical acupuncturists could de-radicalise their claims without fear of losing their distinctiveness. In the eyes of their orthodox medical colleagues, the less distinctive, and the more like orthodox medicine they were, the better. Medical acupuncturists were already doctors and already had access to the benefits given to other medical practitioners. The chiropractors, however, had to argue that they were distinct from the medical profession in order to gain access to those benefits. If they had not been distinct, then there would have been no need to recognise them.

In the analysis of the newsletters and journals, the ebb and flow in the attitudes of the medical acupuncturists are apparent. The irrational could be embraced on one page, and acupuncture could be subordinated to the principles of medical science on another. However, it is an oversimplification to suggest that there is a straightforward dualism here between Western medicine and TCM (Cai 1988). There is a plurality of positions taken up in these debates. The description above belies the notion that we can represent a group by what they say and how they say it in any one forum. The case of medical acupuncturists alerts us to the varieties of presentation and the many sources of tension and conflict within a specific therapeutic practice that leads to particular arguments being presented.

Concluding comments

This chapter has explored a very broad range of influences on therapeutic practices, looking at the state, professional organisation, educational systems and clinical practices through to the everyday practices in the domestic realm. In previous chapters, many features limiting therapeutic pluralism have been outlined, such as regulation by the state, the disciplinary practices of standardisation in education and research and the power of the established medical profession to obstruct opportunities for competing therapeutic modalities. In this chapter, we encounter all these again. However, we also encounter something different. The case of Chinese medicine in China provides a glimpse into the possibilities of state support for therapeutic pluralism, for all the chequered history to the status that Chinese medicine has been given. These opportunities still come with a cost to the therapeutic possibilities of Chinese medicine and have reshaped the forms of that approach. But this re-shaping is inevitable with the transformation of therapeutic practices being a constant. We see this inside China, and when Chinese medicine goes West. The role of nationalism in either subjugating or promoting traditional medicine will be seen in the next chapter as well, when we look at a more complex picture of therapeutic interrelationships on the Indian subcontinent.

In the last chapter, the discursive presentations of orthodox medicine and the heterodox practices of chiropractic were examined, where the polarities of the conflict were transparent. In this chapter, the examination of the discursive presentations of medical acupuncturists reveals a different and crucial aspect of these representations, the situationally specific nature of them. When medical acupuncturist talked to their orthodox medical colleagues, they presented a picture of acupuncture as scientific and as complementary to medicine, but when medical acupuncturists talked amongst themselves about their practices they could claim science, but they could claim many other bases for their practices and express the need to learn from lay practitioners and their more in-depth engagement with Chinese medicine. This examination shows us that not only are therapeutic practices dynamic and constantly evolving, but also they can be multiply represented, and cannot be tied down to one particular understanding of what the world is like and how we can know it and how we can intervene to support health and well-being. On the one hand, we may discern a kind of attenuated pluralism in the way in which Chinese medicine may be taught and researched in Western institutions, but on the other hand, the concept of pluralism is itself open for debate as there is not one entity called Chinese medicine, there are plural TCMs. The multiplicity of therapeutic approaches is omnipresent, and so there are no singular and static systems to which a plural can be contrasted. A further exploration of this incredibly dynamic nature of therapeutic practices occurs in the following chapter.

References

Almeida, J. (2012) The differential incorporation of CAM into the medical establishment: The case of acupuncture and homeopathy in Portugal, *Health Sociology Review*, 765–792.

Baer, H. (2001) *Biomedicine and alternative healing systems in America: Issues of class, race, ethnicity and gender*, Madison: The University of Wisconsin Press.

Barnes, L.L. (2005) *Needles, herbs, gods, and ghosts China, healing, and the West to 1848*, Cambridge, MA: Harvard University Press.

Berliner, H. (1984) Scientific medicine since Flexner, in J.W. Salmon (ed.), *Alternative medicines: Popular and policy perspectives*, New York: Tavistock Press, pp. 30–56.

Bivins, R. (2007) *Alternative medicine: A history*, Oxford: Oxford University Press.

Bowers, J. (1974) American private aid at its peak: Peking Union Medical College, in J. Bowers and E. Purcell (eds.), *Medicine and society in China*, New York: Josiah Macy Jr. Foundation, pp. 82–98.

Bridgman, R. (1974) Traditional Chinese medicine, in J. Bowers and E. Purcell (eds.), *Medicine and society in China*, New York: Josiah Macy Jr. Foundation, pp. 1–21.

Brown Bullock, M. (1974) A brief sketch of the role of the PUMC graduates in the People's Republic of China, in J. Bowers and E. Purcell (eds.), *Medicine and society in China*, New York: Josiah Macy Jr. Foundation, pp. 99–101.

Cai, J. (1988) Integration of traditional Chinese medicine with Western medicine: Right or wrong?, *Social Science and Medicine*, 27, 521–529.

Chow, E.P.Y. (1984) Traditional Chinese medicine: A holistic system, in J.W. Salmon (ed.), *Alternative medicines: Popular and policy perspectives*, New York: Tavistock.

Cohen, P. (1974) Discussion, in J. Bowers and E. Purcell (eds.), *Medicine and society in China*, New York: Josiah Macy Jr. Foundation, pp. 75–81.

Cullen, C. (1993) Patients and healers in later imperial China: Evidence from the Jinpingmei, *History of Science*, 2, 92, 99–150.

Dew, K. (2000) Deviant insiders: Medical acupuncturists in New Zealand, *Social Science & Medicine*, 50, 12, 1785–1795.

——— (2003) *Borderland practices: Regulating alternative therapies in New Zealand*, Dunedin: University of Otago Press.

——— (2012) *The cult and science of public health: A sociological investigation*, London and New York: Berghahn.

Dowson, D. (1985, December) Setting up a clinical trial, *New Zealand Journal of Acupuncture*, 29.

Farquhar, J. (1992) Time and text: Approaching Chinese medical practice through analysis of a published case, in C. Leslie and A. Young (eds.), *Paths to Asian medical knowledge*, Berkeley and Los Angeles: University of California Press, pp. 62–73.

——— (1994) *Knowing practice: The clinical encounter of Chinese medicine*, Boulder: Westview Press.

Frank, R. and Stollberg, G. (2004) Medical acupuncture in Germany: Patterns of consumerism among physicians and patients, *Sociology of Health & Illness*, 26, 3, 351–372.

Freund, P. and McGuire, M. (1991) *Health, illness, and the social body: A critical sociology*, Englewood Cliffs, NJ: Prentice Hall.

Gluckman, L. (1973) Acupuncture, *New Zealand Medical Journal*, 78, 500, 323–325.

Hsu, E. (2001) Figuratively speaking of 'danger in death' in Chinese pulse diagnostics, in R. Jütte, M. Eklöf and M. Nelson (eds.), *Historical aspects of unconventional medicine: Approaches, concepts, case studies*, Sheffield: European Association for the History of Medicine and Health Publications, pp. 193–210.

Kaptchuk, T. (1983) *The web that has no weaver: Understanding Chinese medicine*, New York: Congdon & Weed.

Koplan, J.P., Hinman, A.R., Parker, R.L., Gong, Y.L. and Yang, M.D. (1985) The barefoot doctor: Shanghai county revisited, *American Journal of Public Health*, 75, 7, 768–770.

Lee, S. (1997) WHO and the developing world: The contest for ideology, in A. Cunningham and B. Andrews (eds.), *Western medicine and contested knowledge*, Manchester and New York: Manchester University Press, pp. 24–45.

Leung, B. (2008) *Traditional Chinese medicine: The human dimension*, Sydney: Verdant House.

Malloch, J. (1984) Acupuncture, *New Zealand Medical Journal*, 97, 752, 200–201.

Nathan, C. (1974) The acceptance of Western medicine in early twentieth century China: The story of the North Manchurian Plague Prevention Service, in J. Bowers and E. Purcell (eds.), *Medicine and society in China*, New York: Josiah Macy Jr. Foundation, pp. 55–75.

New Zealand Medical Journal (1982) News from the divisions: Auckland, *New Zealand Medical Journal*, 95, 709, 394.

Ooi, G.I. (1991) The persistence of Chinese medicine: Adjustment and adversity, *Social Science & Medicine*, 32, 3, 261–266.

Porter, T. (1995) *Trust in numbers: The pursuit of objectivity in science and public life*, Princeton: Princeton University Press.

Possamai-Inesedy, A. and Cochrane, S. (2013) The consequences of integrating complementary and alternative medicine: An analysis of impacts on practice, *Health Sociology Review*, 22, 1, 65–74.

Quah, S. (2008) Epilogue: In pursuit of health: Pragmatic acculturation in everyday life, *Health Sociology Review*, 17, 4, 419–422.

Sagli, G. (2001) Chinese medical concepts in biomedical culture: The case of acupuncture in Norway, in R. Jütte, M. Eklöf and M. Nelson (eds.), *Historical aspects of unconventional medicine: Approaches, concepts and case studies*, Sheffield: European Association for the History of Medicine and Health Publications, pp. 211–226.

Saks, M. (1995) *Professions and the public interest: Medical power, altruism and alternative medicine*, London: Routledge.

Scheid, V. (2002) *Chinese medicine in contemporary China: Plurality and synthesis*, Durham, NC: Duke University Press.

Scott, J.C. (1998) *Seeing like a state: How certain schemes to improve the human condition have failed*, New Haven and London: Yale University Press.

Seaman, G. (1992) Winds, waters, seeds and souls: Folk concepts of physiology and etiology in Chinese geomancy, in C. Leslie and A. Young (eds.), *Paths to Asian medical knowledge*, Berkeley: University of California Press, pp. 74–97.

Sidel, R. (1983) *The health of China*, London: Zed.

Sidel, V. (1974) Health services in the People's Republic of China, in J. Bowers and E. Purcell (eds.), *Medicine and society in China*, New York: Josiah Macy Jr. Foundation, pp. 103–127.

Steeper, D. (1985, December) Editorial, *New Zealand Journal of Acupuncture*, 2–3.

Tseung, Y. (1975) Acupuncture, *New Zealand Medical Journal*, 82, 549, 278.

Unschuld, P. (1992) Epistemological issues and changing legitimation: Traditional Chinese medicine in the twentieth century, in C. Leslie and A. Young (eds.), *Paths to Asian medical knowledge*, Berkeley and Los Angeles: University of California Press, pp. 44–61.

Weiss, G. and Lonnquist, L. (2012) *The sociology of health, healing and illness* (7th ed.), Upper Saddle River, NJ: Prentice Hall.

Wolpe, P. (1985) The maintenance of professional authority: Acupuncture and the American physician, *Social Problems*, 32, 5, 409–424.

Wong, G. (1991) Acupuncture therapy: Holistic or symptomatic?, *New Zealand Journal of Acupuncture*, 1991, 2.

6

EMPIRE, TRADITION AND THE MANY THERAPEUTIC FACES OF INDIA

Therapeutic pluralism perhaps fits most comfortably as a descriptor of therapeutic practices in the Indian subcontinent. The relationship between different therapeutic modalities is quite different in India than it is in the West. From the patient perspective, and depending on where in India they live, a number of legitimised modalities are available to choose from, including ayurveda, unani, siddha, homeopathy, Gandhian nature cure and Western biomedicine (Weiss 2009). The first three in this list have been described as 'classical' modalities, but, in precolonial India, they were therapeutic practices that served the elite only (Attewell et al. 2012). Folk medicine or subaltern therapeutic practices served much of the population.

It is also through the social scientific examination of therapeutic activities in this part of the world that the concepts of statist medicine and subaltern therapeutic practices have been developed. The term subaltern therapeutics has been taken up by South-Asian social science scholars to describe those everyday practices, sometimes labelled 'folk medicine', that evade and distance themselves from 'statist medicine' (Hardiman and Mukharji 2012b). My use of statist medicine refers to both the practices of conventional medicine or biomedicine and the state regulatory apparatus in which it is embedded, including the legal requirements around diagnosis, prescription, medical claims-making, market approval and state subsidisation of medicines. In the context of the Indian subcontinent, statist medicine can include ayurveda, unani and siddha traditional practices (and as discussed later, the use of traditional should not be seen as something static and fully formed but evolves and transforms through time and across different spaces). When placed in a Western context, these practices would not be a part of statist medicine. Another important feature of therapeutic pluralism in the Indian subcontinent is the impact of colonialism and imperialism.

Historians have argued that biomedicine or Western medicine is intimately connected with the project of imperialism, to such an extent that Western medicine is imperialist 'as a form of knowledge and as a practice' (Cunningham and Andrews 1997: 1). Medicine was seen by early missionaries as a gateway to both Christianity and trade, and the imposition of Western medicine was a grand act of cultural condescension through dismissing local knowledge (Cunningham and Andrews 1997). However, there are many similarities between Indian, Chinese and pre-biomedical Western scholastic medicine, where the body is conceived as a 'largely fluid entity in dynamic equilibrium . . . endowed with vital energy' (Bivins 2007: 26). Major differences emerge in the seventeenth and eighteenth centuries as Western medicine becomes grounded in anatomy. A new authority based on anatomy fosters scepticism in the West about non-anatomy societies such as India, where dealing with the dead was viewed as polluting, and China, where ancestor worship discourages anatomical dissection (Bivins 2007).

The changing face of Indian therapeutics

The term ayurveda references the idea of a science of life and can be translated as long life (Langford 2002). In ayurveda, life is conceived of as four parts – the soul, the mind, the senses and the body – and these need to be in balance (Islam 2012). Additionally, the three humours of the body, wind, bile and phlegm, known as dosas, need to be in balance to attain health (Obeyesekere 1992). Although referring to many healing practices ayurveda today is associated with three major Sanskrit texts, one focused on surgical treatments and the others on a range of herbal and mineral preparations and a range of techniques such as the use of massage, enemas and bloodletting (Langford 2002). For many, a defining conceptual difference between Western medicine and ayurveda is that the former has an objective or material underpinning, where bodies and diseases are objects, but for ayurveda it has a more dynamic and energetic underpinning, where bodies and diseases are seen in terms of processes and patterns (Langford 2002), similar then to the underpinnings of Chinese medicine discussed in Chapter 5.

In contemporary India, biomedicine could be placed at the top of the medical hierarchy in terms of state support, and since 1995, a department of AYUSH (ayurveda, yoga, unani, siddha, homeopathy, naturopathy and sowa rigpa) was established under the oversight of the Ministry of Health and Family Welfare (Hardiman and Mukharji 2012a). Unani (also known as unani tibb, yunani and tibbia) arrived in India in the seventh century in tow with the political presence of Islam (Berger 2013). Unani medicine, popular in South Asia, is derived from ancient Greek practices and uses humoral theory in diagnosis and treatment. Sowa rigpa is Tibetan medicine, and siddha is a medical tradition from Tamil Nadu, which is discussed later.

In contrast to these clearly identifiable and systematised modalities that have, to various levels, been sanctioned by the state, Guy Attewell et al. (2012) identify subaltern therapeutic practices as a commonly accessed therapeutic dimension. In

India, subaltern therapeutics takes many forms, including the use of allopathy by unqualified healers, bonesetting and massage, mantras and charms disseminated by religious mendicants, the use of divination, plant and animal-based medicines, exorcisms and rituals by a range of unregulated healers, and the provision of treatment for women, particularly pregnant women, by Dais or midwives (Attewell et al. 2012). Subaltern therapeutics can overlap significantly with lay, domestic or household therapeutic practices and health practices embedded in everyday life.

Of the AYUSH systems, homeopathy perhaps stands out as an unusual inclusion. How is it that homeopathy gained such a respectable foothold in Indian therapeutics? Homeopathy arrived in India in the mid-nineteenth century, finding a receptive climate as it was picked up by the *bhadralok* or respectable people (Bivins 2007). Homeopathic hospitals were established by the 1850s, which could be viewed as both modern and Western, but were distanced from imperialism and the hegemonic efforts of Western or allopathic medicine. Homeopathy was seen as neither opposing Indian culture and medicine nor as having a strong association with the insensitivities of imperial medicine.

Infrastructural, technological and economic developments transform therapeutic relations. In the early twentieth century, Hindi, and the Devanagri script, gained dominance in oral and print communication over Urdu. Alongside the expansion of commercial publishing at this time, medical texts were translated into Hindi from other vernaculars, such as Bengali. These developments in publishing also led to a change in medical authority, with information about ayurveda provided by authors who were not trained Brahman vaids who had elite access to ayurvedic knowledge via their understanding of Sanskrit. With the opening up of the public sphere, the practitioner, and not the pandit, became the 'arbiter of tradition' (Berger 2013: 82). The writings of the practitioners did more than transmit the medical knowing of ayurveda, but positioned ayurveda as a legitimate indigenous Indian science, and in so doing was one means for the social reconstruction of Indian identity (Berger 2013).

Sowa Rigpa in Ladakh illustrates changes in practice resulting from economic development. Ladakh is a remote region of India. Practitioners of Sowa Rigpa, known as amchi, had exchange-based social arrangements in the mid-twentieth century that allowed them to practice. These practitioners did not take much in the way of money from their clientele, but people would help the family of the amchi out by assisting with ploughing and harvesting, allowing the amchi the time to practice (Blaikie 2018). Being an amchi was not a full-time occupation but undertaken alongside other work.

The opening up of this remote area through the roading system changed the practices and the role of the amchi. Prior to infrastructural developments, practitioners of Sowa Rigpa had to make up their own medications from locally sourced materials. The materials available may have been more limited than in the post-road era, but the practitioners claimed a deep knowledge of what they were working with (Blaikie 2018). Monks returning from trips to places like

Tibet and Nepal could bring back plant material and gift them to amchi, reinforcing the reciprocity of relationships around healing practices. The post-road era opened up accessibility to a wider range of materials and provided greater opportunities for commercially produced medicines to circulate. The growing influence of pharmacists further facilitated commercialisation over the 2000s, and these developments entwined with efforts to professionalise Sowa Rigpa and have it legitimated, the latter reaching a milestone in 2010 when Sowa Rigpa was recognised by the Indian government (Blaikie 2018).

This did not eliminate localised practices though, with many amchi continuing to make their own medicines, especially ones sourced from local plants, and this practice was also driven by a desire to better understand the different materials in the medicines they were using. Commercial medicines and the availability of raw materials from further afield did have other impacts though, including an increase in the prescription of more complex and potent medicine. Additionally, the success of sowa rigpa in terms of its uptake has put strain on its capacity to meet demand as wild plant sources of medicine become depleted (Blaikie 2018).

The example of sowa rigpa demonstrates how therapeutic practices can be transformed in response to the opportunities and constraints from infrastructural developments. Transformations do occur across therapeutic divides as well. The great traditions of medicine in India, ayurveda, unani and siddha, were not opposed to assimilating aspects of Western medicine into their systems and ways of thinking. For example, germ theory was not seen as incompatible with Indian medicine (Bivins 2007). Ayurveda had a concept of germ causation, but germs were not given the same prominence as causative agents as had occurred in Western medicine. The 'soil' of the body could be as important as the 'seed' of the germ (Bivins 2007). Classical Sanskrit ayurvedic texts incorporated a variety of therapeutic practices, including surgery. The role of surgery in ayurveda disappeared under Brahmanical influence (Lambert 2012). In the early eighteenth century, Indian physicians were happy to combine 'cosmopolitan' medicine introduced by the English and others, and indigenous health practices (Leslie 1992). Ayurveda could also be combined with other systems, such as unani tibb (Leslie 1992).

The therapeutic practices of the Indian subcontinent are not static but take on new forms and different shapes in response to surrounding environmental, political, social and commercial influences. The sources of legitimacy of the various therapeutic modalities differ. The forms of unani and ayurvedic medicine incorporated into AYUSH are more circumscribed than in pre-colonial times with, for example, urine analysis now a marginalised approach (Hardiman and Mukharji 2012a). But Jean Langford (2002: 7) argues that with the colonial impact of European medicine 'ayurveda was gradually transformed from an eclectic set of healing practices to a quintessentially Indian medicine'.

Helen Lambert argues that in Rajasthan Western medicine has not replaced other healing practices, such as ayurveda, unani and a variety of practitioners in rural areas that may use specific approaches such as herbal medicine, bonesetting and divination, but instead Western medicine has added to the plural character of medical practices (Lambert 1997). Villagers position themselves as inexpert in understandings of medicine and disease and their evaluations of therapeutic practices is based on perceived effectiveness, allowing new forms to be taken up on that basis (Lambert 1997), but villagers divide up classes of illness into physician's illness and deity's illness, and so who help is sought from is dependent on the categorisation of the illness (Lambert 1997). Economic factors could also dictate decisions about health seeking, and as seeking the help of a deity through religious ritual was cheaper than the costs of travel and drugs for biomedical treatment then attending a shrine might be the preferred option (Lambert 1997). Therapeutic pluralism is then unevenly spread with those living in rural areas having more limited access to elite therapeutic systems. For those with more wealth, the social prestige of attending the biomedical practitioners with his or her symbolic capital values of modernity might be preferred (Lambert 1997). This choice can play out in gendered ways with women and girl children less likely to be given access to biomedical care (Lambert 1997).

However, the epistemological foundations of biomedicine are not necessarily taken on board by those who attend biomedical practitioners as an indigenous therapeutic framework may be applied. For example, the drugs taken may be seen in the light of humoral theory as having a heating effect, and so might have to be balanced with the consumption of cooling foods (Lambert 1997). Drugs may be seen as a way to quickly alleviate symptoms, but indigenous therapeutics may be required to achieve cure, so biomedicine is not rated as superior to indigenous medicine. In fact unlike indigenous therapy, biomedicine is regarded as having iatrogenic outcomes that would need correction (Lambert 1997). Lambert suggests, based on her observations of the use of Western medicine in Rajasthan, that 'traditional' cultures can be very receptive to new therapeutic systems, but that the new systems or practices may not challenge the underlying therapeutic understandings of these cultures (Lambert 1997).

Changing state support for traditional therapeutics

Several phases of the relationship between European biomedicine and Indian traditional medicine have been suggested and these relationships are politically shaped. During the early stages of colonisation, ayurvedic practitioners could serve as consultants to officials of the East India Company and efforts were made to investigate local medicine and texts for their potential value. In the early nineteenth century phase of colonisation, as it was not possible for Western medicine to support the health care of the Indian population, the colonial administration supported schools to train Indian doctors where biomedicine was taught alongside ayurvedic medicine. In 1822, a new school of medical education was proposed in Calcutta. The manifest goal of this training was to enable Indians to serve the medical needs of the British, but a latent goal was that through the presentation of allopathy alongside traditional medicine the superiority of the former would become apparent, and in turn that would reinforce the superiority of the British race in the eyes of the Indian population (Weiss 2009).

A variation in this relationship between Western medicine and traditional medicine in the early nineteenth century in India was a view that Indian practitioners could be trained via a government supported Native Medical Institution to perform 'sub-duties of European biomedical doctors' at much lower cost (Berger 2013). This hybrid system allowed for the Indian practitioners to continue with their practices whilst undertaking useful labour for the government. This view was not long lived, and a more standardised government-supported education for Indian and European practitioners took hold from 1835. Ayurveda was then excluded from this anglicised form of education (Berger 2013). But at various times through the nineteenth and twentieth century, local Indian practitioners, even those who practiced ayurveda, known as vaids, would be called upon by the Raj and the government to support public health campaigns, especially vaccination campaigns (Berger 2013). The government was then able to utilise these practitioners because of their trusted position in the community to facilitate public health campaigns that might not, in themselves, be trusted.

In India, efforts in the 1860s were made by the colonial authorities to have Western medical practitioners only in government-sponsored programmes, but because of a lack of resources and a lack of political desire this was not achieved (Kumar 1997). In response to this situation in the Punjab native hakims, practitioners of unani were trained in allopathic medicine. The instigator of this scheme hoped that it would subvert the unani system practiced by the hakims as they took on board Western medical ways (Kumar 1997). Such initiatives met with opposition from the government and by the 1880s indigenous Indian practitioners had very little presence in government medical services (Kumar 1997). Even Indians trained in Europe were held in suspicion as it was thought that they would revert to their traditional treatments (Kumar 1997). The imperial government could then shift readily between dismissing ayurveda and unani as irrelevant and unscientific and, in a pragmatic vein, calling upon vaids and hakims and the goodwill they had to undertake certain tasks. For example, in the 1910s, government codes and practices were developed to validate allopathic dispensaries and exclude ayurvedic ones, but the negative impact of closing down all ayurvedic dispensaries was strongly resisted because of their public health campaign role.

Legislation in the early 1900s in India established the Indian Medical Council which excluded practitioners of Indian medicine, and the legislation could be used to remove practitioners of Western medicine who associated with these excluded practitioners (Bivins 2007). However, control of the medical profession was not well institutionalised as it was of little consequence to a practitioner whether they were sanctioned as official medical practitioners or not. Ayurvedic training then shifted to Sanskrit colleges but these colleges adopted some of the institutional practices of Western medicine.

Efforts to revive traditional medicine in the face of unfavourable legislation led in 1910 to the first All India Ayurvedic and Tibbia (Yunani) Conference being organised, which became an annual event. The popularity of such events stimulated a reaction from the colonial government, which in 1912 passed an act excluding indigenous systems from state patronage (Kumar 1997). At the time of the passing of this act, ninety percent of the population used indigenous practitioners, with a widespread revival of ayurveda at the end of the nineteenth century (Kumar 1997). Lobbying of the Indian government led to some appeasement measures, such as the establishment of some tibbia colleges. In 1916, a tibbia college in Delhi was established that had ayurvedic and yunani departments as well as a chemical laboratory and an allopathic section (Kumar 1997). Other colleges of ayurveda education included training in surgery and anatomy (Kumar 1997).

This form of training based on European university models was quite distinct from the extant training of traditional practitioners. Although centres of medical learning were known as far back as the sixth century BC, however, up into the twentieth century many practitioners learnt their skills in small residential centres from one or two gurus, participating in treating patients alongside the gurus for five to seven years (Langford 2002).

Over the twentieth century, the critique of ayurvedic medicine by the British colonisers changed in orientation. Prior to the 1920s, ayurveda was written off as a theoretically outdated system, but with a developing agenda by provincial governments to support indigenous medical systems the critique of ayurveda focused on the substandard training and education of ayurveda practitioners, as well as the poor state of the infrastructure in which the education of practitioners occurred (Berger 2013). In 1921, a Board of Indian Medicine was formed, and an early task of the Board was to register vaids and hakims who could produce government certificates used for sick leave and other purposes. Initially, the registering was ad hoc and based on the perceived reputation of the practitioners and their training (Berger 2013). Vaids and hakims were then drawn into the social control aspects of medicine, and this provided impetus to the professionalisation of ayurvedic medicine. With the Congress winning provincial elections in the United Provinces in 1937, there was a further shift in that ayurveda, as an indigenous system of healing, was viewed as a modality that should be invested in.

Unani practitioners embarked on processes of professional standardisation as early as the 1880s, but ayurveda continued to operate under the guru-Shishya model, beginning to change to more standardised processes of training in the 1920s. The guru model relied on the competence of the teacher, but from the 1920s there was a shift to an education system based on a university model. In response to a disregard of ayurveda, efforts were made to package it in a more standard, or Western, educational form, even by those promoting ayurveda as a part of a nationalist agenda (Langford 2002). But this standardisation was not total. Whereas examination processes for example might follow the forms of Western education, the lineage of gurus was preserved in the particularity of the teaching.

A carrot to induce such a shift to regulated medical education that included allopathy as well as ayurveda was access to positions providing services to government servants. The Board of Indian Medicine provided financial support to colleges of medical education that had a secular and communal vision, promoting a mix of vaids and hakims on the Board of Directors, but this vision did not always align with those promoting ayurveda as a moral system embedded in sacred Sanskrit texts (Berger 2013). It was not until 1976 that a standard modern curriculum was introduced. The shift in teaching style would appear to mean the end of the special relationship between the guru and students based on a close bond as well as a stance of reverence from the students where the guru's teachings were absorbed and knowledge was passed on (Langford 2002). However, in rural areas, training continued under the guru-Shishya model.

In the post-independence environment, there developed a desire to rationalise ayurveda and unani into one system, a task set for the Chopra Report of 1948 to consider. The Chopra Report was a report of the Committee of Indigenous Systems of Medicine. This rationalisation desire was based on the notion that science was universal. In the Chopra Report, the ayurvedic system is regarded as the 'remote source' of Western medicine due to its purported influence on Greek and Arabian medicine (Berger 2013: 164). That is, the claims here for ayurveda are akin to the claims made for siddha medicine, noted later. Unani, on the other hand, was positioned as a recent import (only 1200 years or so ago) arising from the influence of Islam and grounded in the Greek and Arabian traditions that had their sources in ayurveda.

For the state, there were economic reasons for supporting indigenous medicine. In the 1950s, Indigenous dispensaries were favoured by the governments as they were cheaper to operate than allopathic dispensaries, not requiring expensive equipment and using medical ingredients locally sourced (Berger 2013). Through the latter part of the nineteenth century and the early part of the twentieth century, there is then a shift in the conceptualisation of ayurveda by the Government of India from an unscientific modality grounded in mysticism to a set of practices based on knowledge applicable to contemporary times. However, in addition, ayurveda comes under the purview of the state and so becomes a more governable system (Berger 2013).

The revival of ayurvedic educational institutions does not necessarily translate into the promulgation of its practices. Langford notes that in training hospitals ayurvedic students are taught ayurvedic theory in the classroom, but in the wards biomedical disease categories are used when prescribing, categories not necessarily based on ayurvedic disease understandings. This situation is further complicated by the students' capacity to gain a deep knowledge of ayurveda. Most students in ayurvedic institutions do not have sufficient Sanskrit to read the older ayurvedic texts, and their prior school education which takes a standard science approach, does not prepare them for the different concepts they encounter in ayurvedic colleges or the philosophical underpinnings of ayurveda (Langford 2002).

The slippage between biomedicine and ayurveda is also manifested in research on ayurvedic remedies where biomedical disease categories are used with ayurvedic formulations being applied, but ayurvedic diagnostic categories are not used (Langford 2002). The goal of much of this research within a biomedical paradigm was to isolate the active components of remedies. However, ayurvedic physicians resisted this standardisation of drugs and the effort to extract the active component on the basis that the whole drug should be consumed as other ingredients regulated the effect of the active component (Langford 2002).

Research is also challenged by the limits of current scientific thinking around evidence-based hierarchies, with RCTs being the gold standard, as discussed in Chapter 3. Biomedically standardised disease categories are used, such as a specific measure for hypertension, and all patients with those measures can be given the diagnosis of hypertension and enrolled in trials. However, in ayurveda, patients with hypertension may be treated in very different ways, for example, with biomedical drugs, or remedies aimed at systemic change on a particular dosa, or for some other condition such as anxiety (Langford 2002), For practitioners of ayurveda, an approach that can be taken is that rather than give a remedy for a specific disorder a remedy is given to adjust or influence the patient as a whole, or the body as a system (Langford 2002). So, people with the same condition diagnosed in biomedical terms would not necessarily get the same remedy. However, at a commercial and research level, efforts are made to develop ayurvedic drugs that can be used for treating particular conditions, that is, preparations based on a Western medical model (Langford 2002). Because the standardised disease categories of biomedicine do not map onto the disease categories used in ayurveda, it is not clear that ayurvedic approaches should be assessed in the same way as pharmaceuticals within a biomedical framing.

In the latter part of the twentieth century, Nazrul Islam (2012) suggests a new phase, one of new age orientalism. In this phase, there is the commercialisation of ayurveda and its use as a tourist attraction. Islam provides the example of a Vedic Village established in Kolkata, with well-appointed villas and a range of health professionals on hand to provide medical services. But for most of the wealthy customers who stayed at the Village, which in Islam's study included middle-class Indians and tourists from the United States, the United Kingdom, Spain, and the United Arab Emirates, they attended for purposes of relaxation and rejuvenation. Islam suggests that the services on offer were a selection of appealing approaches that romanticised Vedic texts. Massage and yoga could be part of the daily routines but there was scant regard, for example, to the utilisation of seasonal practices as outlined in Vedic texts (Islam 2012).

Into the twenty-first century, there have been further developments in the commercialising of Indian traditional therapeutic approaches captured in the term 'yogapreneurism' (Misra 2017). A very successful example of a yogapreneur is Baba Ramdev. Baba Ramdev is a well-known advocate of traditional medicine in India (Khalikova 2017). Through his television broadcasts as a tele-guru, he has attracted an estimated eighty-five million followers in many countries. He co-founded a business network called Patanjali Ayurvedic Limited that includes an ayurveda pharmaceutical company, hospitals, a publishing house, yoga retreats and food manufacturing (Khalikova 2017). Although espousing asceticism Venera Khalikova argues that Baba Ramdev represents a turn from asceticism to biomoral consumerism, with consumption pivoting around concerns about national identify. It is through yoga and ayurveda that prestige will be restored to India. The consumption of homegrown medicine, as well as other purportedly healthier alternatives to the goods sold by multinational companies, such as noodles, ketchup and toothpaste, promotes a physically healthy population and strengthens the Indian economy.

Enacting traditional practices

The ebb and flow of the credibility given to and the legitimation of traditional practices at the legislative and political level belie the ongoing therapeutic activities of traditional approaches in the everyday. The relationship between biomedicine and alternative therapeutics is quite different in India than it is in most Western countries. The use of everyday items for medicinal purposes, such as turmeric and cumin, is something that people may be brought up with, so that they are practicing traditional medical approaches before they are aware of therapeutic distinctions (Broom et al. 2009)

One important principle of ayurveda is the interconnection of the humours, or dosas, of which there are three, wind, bile and phlegm. The task of the vaidya is to balance the dosas, which may require calming them through dietary and pharmacological means. According to ayurvedic writings, a diagnosis incorporates issues of regional ecology, the season, the weather and a person's constitution (Leslie 1992). This complex form of diagnosis can contrast with the claims made in much Western sociological critiques of CAM practices that it individualises illness and disease as the patient being responsible for cause and the effects of treatment. In this reading of the ayurvedic tradition, the practitioner 'displaces' responsibility from the individual, finding cause in the complicated interactions of humours, bodily constitution, seasonal states and so on (Leslie 1992).

In early twentieth-century medical books in India, the idea that local medicines were required for local illnesses was articulated, and this was based on a view that people had different constitutions that related to climate, geography and local flora. This view was extended to take in different religious constitutions with unani therapeutics being appropriate for Muslim bodies, but not appropriate for Hindu bodies (Berger 2013). This concept could be used to resist the encroachment of Western medicine on health grounds, that is, Western medicine is good for Europeans but will not be good for the Indian population (Langford 2002).

Ayurveda is also enacted differently resulting from varying responses to its elite religious foundation. Ayurvedic medicine has different nuances in different geographical and social contexts. Ayurveda in Sri Lanka can be interpreted in a way that rejects its Brahmanic stories of mythic foundations, and instead can be seen as a pragmatic therapeutic practice, not bound down to theory (Obeyesekere

1992). These complex relationships play out for other prominent traditions on the Indian subcontinent, such as siddha medicine to which we now turn.

Nationalism and modernity in the practice of siddha

The example of siddha medicine powerfully illustrates how complex interactions between different modalities occur, the sources of legitimation and the interactions between nationalism and medicine. Siddha is a therapeutic approach, or perhaps a number of therapeutic approaches, that is indigenous to India, with its home in Tamil Nadu.

Those wanting to receive formal training in siddha today can study for a Bachelor of Siddha Medicine and Surgery at several colleges. As at 2007, there were 275 siddha hospitals and 5051 registered practitioners of siddha medicine in Tamil Nadu, and in comparison, there were 3,612 registered ayurveda practitioners and 1,014 registered unani practitioners in that state (Weiss 2009). However, many more practitioners are not officially recognised, having received a hereditary form of education or apprenticeship.

This traditional practice of siddha operates alongside other forms of traditional practice as well as biomedicine, and in such a competitive marketplace of therapeutic modalities, the knowledge and therapeutics of siddha practitioners must be seen as relevant and effective. For some siddha medical practitioners, a feature of its practice that distinguishes it from ayurveda is the role of alchemy, that is, the transformation of metals, with mercury in particular being a central metal in this process (Weiss 2009). However, the preparation of metals for medical purposes is a costly process and so some practitioners would focus on the use of plant-based medicines. Plant-based or herbal remedies have been written up in self-help books that allow for the domestic use of these preparations. Local ingredients formed the basis of these medicines, aligning with the idea that the cures for disease can be found in the locations where those diseases occur. Other books based in the siddha tradition outline the therapeutic properties of everyday foods in the Tamil cuisine, and that non-Tamil foods can be the cause of illness.

Siddha doctors, vaidyas being the term for practitioners of traditional medicine, trace the origins of their therapeutic practices to a group of extraordinary Tamil medical yogis, called siddhars, who had obtained supernatural powers (Weiss 2009). The siddhars promoted a more egalitarian system than the caste system and rejected the ritualistic approaches of Brahmans (Weiss 2009). The ultimate goal of siddha medicine is to make the body immortal, so that the soul is immortal, based in a cosmology where the soul animates the body but without the body the soul is only steam (Trawick 1992). Siddhars seek a lifeless form through deep trance and other practices that free them from the need for nurture and it is a changeless form. The use of minerals in siddha medicine aligns with this ultimate goal, in that minerals have a lifeless-deathless quality and have the power to cause death through toxicity or restore life (Trawick 1992).

With the moves to what Richard Weiss refers to as an homogenising project of Indian nationalism in the twentieth century, siddha was threatened by the attempt to base a single national system of traditional therapeutic practices on Sanskrit text and ayurvedic practice (Weiss 2009). As such, siddha medicine needed to respond not only to the dismissive stance of biomedicine but also to the challenge of other traditional practices that could engulf it.

In promoting siddha medicine's relevance, and in promoting Tamil nationalism, siddha medicine authorities looked to an ancient past where Tamil knowledge and medical practices pre-dated Sanskrit knowledge. The narrative of the ancient past in Tamil revivalist histories references a prehistoric island called Lemuria, in which a utopian society prevailed, and a medical system operated that could cure any ailment. This perfect society was corrupted following Brahman invasion, one that introduced ayurveda to Tamil society (Weiss 2009). In addition, supporters of siddha suggest that contemporary siddha medicine practices may need to be purged of Sanskritic elements, which have led to its degeneration, so that siddha medicine can potentially be restored to its former glory prior to Aryan influences (Weiss 2009).

Siddha therapeutic practices are based on thousands of palm-leaf manuscripts attributed to one or other of the siddhars, and that were passed down over the centuries, although most that survived are now housed in libraries and archives in Tamil Nadu (Weiss 2009). These manuscripts detail rituals, recipes and practices. Claims are made that the medical system contained in these manuscripts and others that have been corrupted, lost or not yet assembled, contained the work of geniuses who had the scientific sophistication to discern the principles of medicine and health, and that this system was the original medical system of the world (Weiss 2009: 53). In the siddha medical tradition, science reached its apex in the ancient past, but much of its scientific basis has been lost or forgotten. As such, science has been cast as a central element in the tradition of siddha medicine (Weiss 2009), but science can be found in different dimensions of time in siddha (and ayurveda) medicine and Western medicine. For siddha, perfected science has become corrupted and lost, and the current task it to restore ancient knowledge. For Western medicine, progress is to move away from the past and into a future of more advanced knowledge.

Weiss (2009) argues that it is only in the twentieth century that the idea of a unified Tamil medical tradition was imagined, as siddha medicine was based on hereditary lineages where vaidyas traced their particular practices back to a founding siddhar. Knowledge and practice were passed on, but often surrounded in secrecy and mystery. This hereditary form of knowledge transfer persists today and is in tension with efforts to systematise siddha medical practice and so standardise siddha medicine education. Knowledge was transmitted from guru to student, with medical formulae varying down the different lines of transmission. Thus, transmission of knowledge was controlled, and formulae could be concealed from those not initiated. In contemporary times, in order to make these medicines available for the good of the whole Tamil community, calls have been made for the state to compensate siddhas for their medical formulae, so that they could be made public (Weiss 2009).

Hereditary forms of transmission are also in tension with efforts to develop and innovate and respond to new diseases and conditions. To innovate is to go beyond a traditional teaching, and these teachings need to be preserved and not contaminated or tampered with. To tamper with a traditional teaching is to corrupt it and add in imperfections to a perfect system. A position can be taken then that siddha medicine and other traditional Indian medicines may be in a state of decay due to foreign influences, so what is required is a process of purification (Weiss 2009). For siddha medical practitioners trained within a hereditary system, the college-trained siddha practitioners have become corrupted by Western traditions (Weiss 2009).

Siddha medicine is also in tension with the universalising claims of Western science. Rhetorically Western biomedical practitioners may claim that there is only one rational system that is based on universal truth, and so there is only one science, but in siddha medicine there is Western science and Tamil science. Vaidyas see Tamil science as predating Western science, and it is a more profound science as it goes beyond consideration of the physical and material world to consider the divine, which manifests in physical substances, and as such, its standards of assessment and its assumptions and values may be incommensurable with Western science. Tamil science is a rational science, not one based on superstition and ritual, but one that has become corrupted by Brahmanic cultural forms, and can, sometime in the future, be fully regained (Weiss 2009).

The skills of the vaidyas may also differ from the requirement of a Western medical education. For siddha practitioners, the body can be divided into the gross physical body, which is the primary domain of biomedicine, and a subtle body which one gains insights into through intuition and spiritual insights (Weiss 2009). Another dimension of siddha medicine, that, as mentioned, is also claimed by other Indian therapeutic modalities and that challenges universalising practices, is a view that local medicines are best used for treating local diseases and bodies. One basis for this view is a humoral theory of health and disease that siddha (along with ayurveda and unani medicine) draws on. The humours of wind, bile and phlegm need to be in balance, and these humours are impacted by environmental factors, such as the climate and the season (Weiss 2009).

For all the tension with ayurveda, siddha medicine vaidyas will work with ayurvedic vaidyas and unani hakims in response to the incursions of biomedicine and its universalising and standardising projects and imperial connections (Weiss 2009). There is also much overlap in the concepts and practices deployed by siddha and ayurveda practitioners. But traditional practitioners in India are not unified in their response to biomedicine. For example, in 1947, The College of Integrated Medicine was founded in Madras to, as the title suggests, integrate different medical practices, a goal that many practitioners would contest.

Siddha medicine and its trajectory and discursive representations highlight the interplay between different traditional medicines and orthodox medicine and the ways in which therapeutic practices are justified and rationalised in relation to the broader social impact of historical invasion, colonialism and the embracing and resistance to standardising practices. Other forms of practice, here termed subaltern practices, also resist standardising processes.

Subaltern practices

Lambert contests the notion of systems of Indian medicine, rather seeing them as more recent reformulations into discrete 'professional knowledge systems', but still inaccessible to 'large sections of the subaltern population' (Lambert 2012: 110). That is, with the state incorporation of AYUSH large sectors of the population in India remain underserved by official medical services. Furthermore, Lambert argues that the urban and rural poor reject, resist or contest both biomedical conceptions of health and disease and any view of elite medical therapeutics as superior.

There are myriad subaltern practices in the Indian subcontinent. In India, there are what could be described as indigenous healing practices that neither fit with the traditional therapeutic systems of ayurveda, unani tibb and siddha, nor with more recent imports such as allopathy and homeopathy.

The example of chandshir medicine provides detail on some forms in which these practices may take, how they operate, how they may contest Western understandings of knowledge, diagnosis and the healer-patient relationship, and the contingent nature of this. Chandshir medicine is an example of a subaltern therapeutics that appears to sit outside of the classic traditions of South Asian medicine, but is difficult to document and record because of its limited presence in the historical record. Chandshir was a form of medicine based in Bengal and a founding narrative describes the gift of two secret medicines, Gol and Kait, from a Goddess to Bishnuhori Das in 1770, which was then passed down through his descendants and spread out across parts of South Asia (Mukharji 2012). The therapeutic practices of chandshir differ from many therapeutic systems where, for the latter, diagnosis and treatment take place inside private rooms and spaces (hospitals of course operating differently). In chandshir practices, diagnosis can occur in a public reception area, where ex-patients, relatives and friends of the practitioner and patients may be in attendance. Diagnosis is an interactional and conversational event, in which others may enter into the discussion beyond the patient and practitioner. Reference may be made by regulars and the practitioners to other similar cases, and out of this fluid interaction, a diagnosis is arrived at and a treatment agreed to (Mukharji 2012). This kind of process will elude efforts to standardise diagnosis and treatment, as the outcomes are collectively arrived at and variable.

Outside of urban spaces, other forms of healing operate. These are tribal healers, such as the bhagats in South Gujarat. The bhagats are involved in individual illnesses where herbal cures may be used, through to collective illness that may require the propitiation of spirits (Raje 2012). The therapeutic practices of bhagats are based on specialised knowledge of local flora, with the bhagats gathering their own herbs and plants for medical preparation. But this is increasingly challenged due to the loss of forestation where plants would be found, through to the limitation of access to forests, so they could be the preserve of ayurvedic pharmacies (Raje 2012).

Lambert observes that in contemporary times in Rajasthan fractures and dislocations are often treated by bonesetters outside of the formal health sector (Lambert 2012). Bonesetters who reset fractures and dislocations in rural Rajasthan were not formally trained, but often recognised as having a special gift and may treat both livestock and humans. Knowledge of who to go to and what sort of fractures bonesetters are happy to treat is local, and depending on the complaint, a practitioner will be tried out. Many of the local healers, bonesetters and others, practice when needed and do not do therapeutic work for a living, usually refusing remuneration (Lambert 2012).

Another commonly practiced subaltern therapeutic approach that Lambert encountered in Rajasthan was conceptualised as vessel manipulation, where a navel pulse required relocating through physical manipulation. A dislocation could cause a range of symptoms, many seemingly gastrointestinal in nature such as constipation and loss of appetite. Lambert argues that these structures manipulated by local healers have no clear relationship to the bodily structures recognised by biomedical physiology, and so are not amenable to allopathic intervention. She suggests that '[v]essel manipulation thus offers an example of visceral resistance to biomedical hegemony' (Lambert 2012: 122). However, this resistance is all but invisible to state forces as both bonesetting and vessel manipulation have not been positioned within any professionalising strategies and have not been regulated through policy or researched for their therapeutic value (Lambert 2012).

Attempts to revive traditional medicine and subaltern practices to empower people and reduce costs on healthcare systems take different forms, where state practices can actively attempt to cultivate forms of subaltern practice. In 1993, in Bangalore and Tamil Nadu, the Foundation for the Revitalization of Local Health Traditions (FRLHT) was formed, and one initiative they developed was the Home Herbal Garden (HHG) (Hollenberg and Torri 2013) The HHG initiative included such activities as the establishment of a conservation park for medicinal plants (of which thousands have been identified) to educate villagers about these plants and folk healing practices. Community-based enterprises to cultivate and utilise medicinal plants have also been established, and an off-shoot of that activity is an increasingly prominent role played by women as consultants and the enhancement of their social status (Hollenberg and Torri 2013).

Subaltern practices then take a great variety of forms, enacting distinctly different diagnostic and therapeutic practices, and grounded in a plethora of understandings of cause and effect. These practices are rarely legible to the state but are made available as local community practices and evaluated through community understandings.

Conclusion

Kaleidoscopic changes in components between and within therapeutic practices are dramatised in the Indian subcontinent. Responses to colonial administrations and therapeutics can be pragmatic and ideological, and therapeutics can be a site of cultural revival and nationalism. The range of health practices are shaped through engagement with each other, with therapeutic assimilation and contamination occurring alongside efforts at purification, within the purview of the state and beyond it. Alignment between political stances and therapeutics could create sharp divides. Langford notes explicit alliances between politics and therapeutics, providing the example of an ayurvedic practitioner who gave up using tablets and injections in his practice because he wanted to align his practice with his political stance on nationalism and cultural revival (Langford 2002). These therapeutic practices are ever changing in response to ideological, social, political, technological and environmental unfoldings.

Traditional medicine can be positioned for strategic purposes in different ways including as symbolic of national identity, as complementary to biomedicine, and as representing complete healing systems based on eternal truths (Langford 2002). Traditional medicine does not stay the same and responds to biomedicine, as biomedicine responds to traditional therapeutics. There are dynamic interactions between patient, practitioner and competing health systems. In India, with the introduction of biomedicine, patients came to expect the use of injections and antibiotics, and so non-biomedical healers can incorporate these into their practices, and conversely biomedical practitioners respond to patient expectations in prescribing elaborate dietary practices that accompany medical prescriptions (Trawick 1992).

On the surface, therapeutic pluralism abounds at all levels, the state, professional groupings, individual practice and in everyday life. At a nationalist level, there are stark differences in the positioning of science. For siddha and ayurvedic medicine science is to be recovered by removing the contaminations of original understandings that have accrued over the centuries, and for biomedicine science is a process of progress improving on the past. But apart from some subaltern practices, the spectre of biomedical science and the cultural hegemony of Western medicine haunt these different practices.

References

Attewell, G., Hardiman, D., Lambert, H. and Mukharji, P.B. (2012) Agendas, in D. Hardiman and P.B. Mukharji (eds.), *Medical marginality in South Asia: Situating subaltern therapeutics*, London and New York: Routledge, pp. 1–5.

Berger, R. (2013) *Ayurveda made modern: Political histories of indigenous medicine in North India, 1900–1955*, London, UK: Palgrave Macmillan.

Bivins, R. (2007) *Alternative medicine: A history*, Oxford: Oxford University Press.

Blaikie, C. (2018) Absence, abundance, and excess: Substances and Sowa Rigpa in Ladakh since the 1960s, in R.D. Roy and G.N.A. Attewell (eds.), *Locating medicine*, Oxford: Oxford University Press, pp. 169–199.

Broom, A., Doron, A. and Tovey, P. (2009) The inequalities of medical pluralism: Hierarchies of health, the politics of tradition and the economies of care in Indian oncology, *Social Science & Medicine*, 69, 698–706.

Cunningham, A. and Andrews, B. (1997) Introduction: Western medicine as contested knowledge, in A. Cunningham and B. Andrews (eds.), *Western medicine as contested knowledge*, Manchester and New York: Manchester University Press, pp. 1–23.

Hardiman, D. and Mukharji, P.B. (2012a) Introduction, in D. Hardiman and P.B. Mukharji (eds.), *Medical marginality in South Asia: Situating subaltern therapeutics*, London and New York: Routledge, pp. 6–35.

——— (2012b) *Medical marginality in South Asia: Situating subaltern therapeutics*, London: Routledge.

Hollenberg, D. and Torri, M.C. (2013) Linking complementary and alternative medicine, traditional medicine and primary health care: The role of local health traditions in promoting health security, in J. Adams, P. Magin and A. Broom (eds.), *Primary health care and complementary and integrative medicine: Practice and research*, London: Imperial College Press, pp. 93–114.

Islam, N. (2012) New age orientalism: Ayurvedic 'wellness and spa culture', *Health Sociology Review*, 21, 2, 220–231.

Khalikova, V.R. (2017) The ayurveda of Baba Ramdev: Biomoral consumerism, national duty and the biopolitics of 'homegrown' medicine in India, *South Asia: Journal of South Asian Studies*, 40, 1, 105–122.

Kumar, D. (1997) Unequal contenders, uneven ground: Medical encounters in British India, 1820–1920, in A. Cunningham and B. Andrews (eds.), *Western medicine as contested knowledge*, Manchester and New York: Manchester University Press, pp. 172–190.

Lambert, H. (1997) Plural traditions? Folk therapeutics and 'English' medicine in Rajasthan, in A. Cunningham and B. Andrews (eds.), *Western medicine and contested knowledge*, Manchester and New York: Manchester University Press, pp. 191–211.

——— (2012) Wrestling with tradition: Towards a subaltern therapeutics of bonesetting and vessel treatment in north India, in D. Hardiman and P.B. Mukharji (eds.), *Medical marginality in South Asia: Situating subaltern therapeutics*, London and New York: Routledge, pp. 109–125.

Langford, J. (2002) *Fluent bodies: Ayurvedic remedies for postcolonial imbalance*, Durham: Duke University Press.

Leslie, C. (1992) Interpretations of illness: Syncretism in modern ayurveda, in C. Leslie and A. Young (eds.), *Paths to Asian medical knowledge*, Berkeley: University of California Press, pp. 177–208.

Misra, K.R. (2017) 'Yogapreneur' Baba Ramdev and Patanjali Ayurved Limited, *Sectoral Entrepreneurship*, http://library.ediindia.ac.in:8181/xmlui/handle/123456789/5997.

Mukharji, P.B. (2012) Chandshir Chikitsha: A nomadology of subaltern medicine, in D. Hardiman and P.B. Mukharji (eds.), *Medical marginality in South Asia: Situating subaltern therapeutics*, London and New York: Routledge, pp. 85–108.

Obeyesekere, G. (1992) Science, experimentation, and clinical practice in ayurveda, in C. Leslie and A. Young (eds.), *Paths to Asian medicine knowledge*, Berkeley: University of California Press, pp. 160–176.

Raje, G. (2012) The modernising bhagat, in D. Hardiman and P.B. Mukharji (eds.), *Medical marginality in South Asia: Situating subaltern therapeutics*, London and New York: Routledge, pp. 152–170.

Trawick, M. (1992) Death and nurturance in Indian systems of healing, in C. Leslie and A. Young (eds.), *Paths to Asian medical knowledge*, Berkeley: University of California Press, pp. 129–159.

Weiss, R. (2009) *Recipes for immortality medicine, religion, and community in South India*, Oxford: Oxford University Press.

7

THE CAM USER AND THE EXPANSION OF THERAPEUTIC POSSIBILITIES

The etymological sense of the term 'patient' is someone who endures (Hess 2004). This suggests a passive role in a paternalistic system, and indeed in both mainstream medicine and CAM, paternalism is present (Frank and Stollberg 2004). Other terms, like consumer, can suggest a more active role, but also may convey meanings of someone who shops around for what best suits them. Arguably, it is at the level of the individual patient, client, consumer or seeker of health that we can discern an enhanced therapeutic liberty, a little freer from the systemic and structural constraints of statist medicine. But rather than therapeutic pluralism, I suggest that the term therapeutic hybridity captures the practices of CAM and biomedicine in households.

The general public are high consumers of CAM products and services. Studies in Australia, the United Kingdom, Europe, Canada and the United States show that there has been a considerable growth in the popularity of alternative therapies since the 1960s (Saks 2001). In the United States, one in five people consult a CAM practitioner (Harris and Rees 2000). In the United Kingdom, around a quarter of the population use CAM each year and at least one in ten consult a CAM practitioner each year, despite most CAM services requiring out of pocket charges (Sharp et al. 2018). Nearly half the population of English adults are estimated to have used one of the established CAM approaches during their lifetime (Sointu 2012). CAM use is extensive in Australia where health insurance schemes allow widespread access, with over two-thirds of the population reportedly using CAM and forty-four percent having visited a CAM practitioner within the year (Xue et al. 2007), and spending on CAM therapies is greater than spending on prescription drugs (Possamai-Inesedy and Cochrane 2013).

Whatever the precise numbers, and this depends very much on how one defines alternative medicine, a substantial proportion of the population appear to be interested in alternative therapies and alternative medicines, and many practitioners are supported financially by their practices. In this chapter, I will cover some of the major explanations given for why people attend alternative therapists or take non-orthodox remedies. Attempts at providing simple explanations are challenged when we look at the complexity of CAM use by those who use it in their homes, and this will be discussed alongside what can happen when CAM use becomes an issue in orthodox medical practices. But first, the question arises, why do people go to alternative therapists given the prestige, status and resources at the disposal of the orthodox medical profession? There are many suggestions as to why people attend alternative therapists.

Explaining the use of alternative medicines

Dissatisfaction with conventional treatment appears to be a major reason for people seeking alternative medicine. Studies in the United Kingdom, Sweden, Australia and elsewhere have found that between fifty and seventy percent of users of alternative medicine do so because they have not gained relief for their conditions from orthodox medicine or they were dissatisfied with their doctors (Baarts and Pedersen 2009; Lynöe and Svensson 1992; Nicholls 1988; Sharma 1992). This reason for supporting alternative medicine even comes from within the medical profession. New Zealand and Australian studies have found that between sixty and seventy percent of orthodox practitioners who referred patients to alternative therapists did so due to the failure of orthodox treatment to satisfactorily deal with the health problem their patients confronted (Marshall and Gee 1990; Parliament of Victoria Social Development Committee 1986).

Related to this issue of dissatisfaction with orthodox medicine are findings that indicate that users of alternative therapies tend to have chronic conditions. Studies in Britain, Canada and Australia indicate that as many as eighty percent of those consulting complementary therapists do so for chronic musculo-skeletal complaints or other chronic conditions (Clavarino and Yates 1995; Kelner and Wellman 1997; Sharma 1996). The Canadian study also found that, compared to people who consulted only family physicians, those who consulted alternative practitioners were more likely to report their illness or injury as definitely affecting their daily lives, which suggests that the condition is more debilitating or disabling for those who consult alternative therapists.

The concept of the sick role, or an extension of it, can be used to provide insight into the processes at play here. Talcott Parsons, who articulated the concept of the sick role, defines health as 'the state of optimum capacity of an individual for the effective performance of the roles and tasks for which he [*sic*] has been socialized' (Parsons 1958). Therefore, illness is an incapacity of an individual to effectively perform social roles. Parsons identified a number of features of the sick role. One is that recovery depends upon a therapeutic process. In this sense, the patient is not responsible for recovery, but the therapeutic agent is. Illness exempts one from normal role obligations, such as going to work, but this must be seen as undesirable and the patient must try to get well. As part of this, the patient is obliged to seek help from competent agencies. Parsons' perspective appears grounded in the therapeutic efficacy of orthodox medicine. But what happens when orthodox medicine does not work and the patient is in a situation of chronic illness? The health-seeking behaviours we see from many people are that the imperative to seek help in the face of illness does not stop when medicine fails. Many people will seek out other options, and in Parsons' terms this may take the form of an obligation to do so in continuing efforts to get well.

There is some evidence that CAM use may result in decreases in the use of biomedical resources, such as reducing hospital admission and pharmaceutical use (Willison et al. 2013). But the increasing popularity of alternative therapies is unlikely to be a sign of a rejection of the use of orthodox medical services, but as additional to that use. A Canadian study showed that in the period between 1979 and 1988 people utilised alternative therapies more frequently, but there was no decrease in the use of prescription medicine (Northcott and Bachynsky 1993). Those who had consulted alternative therapists are also high attendees at orthodox practices (Murray and Shepherd 1993; Sharma 1992). This is likely to be explained by people who have chronic conditions being high users of healing modalities of any sort.

What the body of research noted here suggests is that people seek out CAM in order to address specific health concerns that orthodox medicine has not been able to satisfactorily address. But do people have a philosophical alignment with CAM? In a study of German patients using medical acupuncture, it was found that none of the patients had an ideological background that would have been a reason for their use of acupuncture (Frank and Stollberg 2004). Patients might come to acupuncture because of a failure of biomedicine to deal with their condition, but this did not mean that biomedicine was rejected outright. Once using acupuncture, none of the patients went on to study it up or learn more about it, rather, they took on the role of passive patients who were leaving their health care in the hand of experts (Frank and Stollberg 2004). This contrasts with some other research that shows patient interest in their therapeutic modalities (Jakes and Kirk 2015), which suggests that there is a range of ways in which patients interact with these modalities that might relate to the modality itself, some characteristic of the patient or of the country in which the treatment is provided, or some other reason. But the German patients were attracted to medical acupuncturists who were able to keep appointment times and provided a quality of service, perhaps as much a characteristic of private care in relation to a public system as it is to the modality (Frank and Stollberg 2004).

As noted in Chapter 3, it is also apparent that very few of those who consult non-orthodox practitioners tell their GPs that they have done so (Steel et al. 2013). Patients feared ridicule or disapproval from their GP and were concerned that the GP would see this as flouting his or her medical authority (Sharma 1992). Patients would not mention their use of CAM because they were not asked about it by their doctors or they did not realise that it was something that they should mention (Penney et al. 2016). Additionally, many people do not consult medical doctors about ailments being treated by a non-conventional therapist (Consumers' Institute 1997).

As opposed to focusing on CAM being additional to orthodox medicine, some theorists consider a cultural change as the reason for the increasing popularity of CAM. CAM use may be a reflection of postmodern values such as the rejection of scientific and professional authority (Siahpush 1998). Some suggest that alternative medicine is a visible sign of the embracing of a new age lifestyle (Coward 1989). This kind of argument is made when the focus is on particular types of therapeutic approach such as the human potential movement, spiritual healing and the use of crystals. This position is in conflict with the research suggesting that people use alternative therapies for pragmatic reasons, and most frequently for musculo-skeletal complaints. Eeva Sointu (2006) notes that people seek out CAM for a host of reasons, from a desperate attempt to find relief in the face of terminal illness to everyday health maintenance, but she places strong emphasis on the place of well-being for patients and practitioners of CAM. Her study focused on middle-class and well-educated women who used a variety of CAM approaches, including rebirthing, shiatsu and yoga. For many, seeking out better health could be articulated as having the goal of 'being fully me' (Sointu 2006: 336). The CAM patient is positioned as knowledgeable and empowered, a much more active role than the passive patient in biomedical framings, or than the acupuncture patients that Robert Frank and Gunnar Stollberg (2004) studied.

In contrast, others suggest that very few people using alternative treatments show an interest in alternative culture, lifestyles or politics, and in fact patients are quite sceptical of non-orthodox medicine before they try it (Sharma 1992). Initial consultations are motivated by pragmatic concerns, and subsequent decisions will be influenced by the outcome of this initial encounter. The patient's beliefs are not necessarily the same as the non-orthodox practitioners, though they may be influenced by the practitioner's beliefs and values during the course of the encounter. For some patients though, an interest in the philosophy can develop with further engagement with treatment (Jakes and Kirk 2015). Canadian research found differences between various therapies, with fewer patients 'believing' in the type of care offered by chiropractors, and a greater number 'believing' in the principles of reiki (Kelner and Wellman 1997). So, variations in clientele between different alternative therapies are as significant as variations between orthodox medicine and alternative medicine. This Canadian study did find that those who consulted alternative practitioners tended to have a greater belief that they were responsible for their healthcare decisions, whereas those who consulted orthodox medicine only tended to view the physician as being responsible for their healthcare decisions. The passive sick role then plays out more clearly in the orthodox consultation than in the consultation with alternative practitioners. Arguably, this supports a view that there has not been any major cultural shift in relation to health beliefs though there may be higher expectations placed on medicine and an increasing importance placed on the cure and care of the body in modern society (Sharma 1996: 231).

People may use CAM during particular events or phases in their lives, for example, women use CAM at a high rate during the period of menopausal transition (Steel et al. 2013). Not surprisingly, there is a link between parents' use of CAM and children's use of CAM. In a US study, a child was five times more likely to have used CAM in the last twelve months if their parents used CAM (Barnes et al. 2008).

Sointu (2012) notes that both clients and CAM practitioners are predominantly women. She suggests that the sphere of CAM, or more specifically in her research, the sphere of holistic health, is gendered. She suggests that the attributes of 'care, empathy and acceptance' (Sointu 2012: 72) are aligned with femininity in contemporary Western culture, and that these attributes are also aligned with holistic healthcare practices. An alternative or complementary reading to this is that many CAM practitioners are in subordinated, part-time positions. CAM practices provide opportunities to have some control over the hours and timing of work, as practitioners are often self-employed. This aligns with the structural position of women in contemporary society who may still have the responsibility and duty of mothering that limits opportunities in many spheres of work.

Sointu further suggests that the holistic practices that were the focus of her research provide, for the clients, a challenge to the traditional family where the mother, as primary carer, puts others before herself. The messages of finding oneself and living to one's potential, and not just being there for others, may be a means of resistance to traditional feminine values (Sointu 2012). Sointu (2012: 136) also refers to holistic health being entwined with 'narcissistic pampering'. These views of CAM are in stark contrast to some other studies that show, for example, the stringent and self-abnegatory practices that some clients take – an issue we will cover in Chapter 8 on cancer and CAM.

Given the diversity of CAM practices, it seems clear that there is no easy generalisation to make about why people use CAM. The reasons for its use are nearly as diverse as the therapeutic offerings available. But a commonly articulated reason for people seeking out unconventional therapies is a pragmatic one, where conventional medicine has not been able to satisfactorily resolve a chronic, often musculoskeletal, problem. People in a position to do this are more likely to have a higher income and a higher education, with evidence of women using these services more than men. Those therapies that have a focus on personal development and fulfilling one's potential may attract a different clientele, and certainly would likely be accessed for different reasons, as we see in Sointu's study. For those seeking CAM help for pragmatic reasons, there is rarely an initial ideological commitment to the philosophy or assumptions of the therapy, but for some who use the therapy over a longer period of time these philosophical underpinnings may become of interest.

Using CAM in the home

Much of CAM use takes place in the home. Over time, there have been shifts in the capacity and the resources available to householders in relation to therapeutic possibilities. For example, David Arnold suggests that the development of the Indian postal service, along with the expansion of advertising and the development of pre-packaged allopathic and ayurvedic medicines as well as self-help homeopathy in India, fostered self-medication practices and reduced a reliance on formal doctoring (Arnold 2018). Across the globe developments in on-line consumerism has enabled much greater access to different therapeutic agents, including CAM ones such as supplements and herbal preparations (Nettleton 2004).

In research undertaken on therapeutic practices in households and in the home, the diversity of practices, and the many different therapeutic modalities and how they are used are starkly revealed (Chamberlain et al. 2011; Dew 2016; Dew et al. 2014; Dew et al. 2015; Hodgetts et al. 2011; Hodgetts et al. 2017). This section draws on research on household therapeutic practices that I conducted with colleagues, where we went into people's homes and explored householders' access to, consumption of and understandings of medications and remedies. It is clear that for many people, when they take advice from biomedical practitioners, from CAM practitioners, from friends, workmates and family members, from the internet and the mass media, they make their own determinations about what to prioritise, who to trust and what to do. People may combine different therapeutic modalities in ways not anticipated by health practitioners sitting in their clinics, and mostly, not even known by these practitioners. People can hybridise different practices (Latour 1993), so that what is kept apart in the consulting rooms of practitioners is put together within the spaces of the home. People do not simply accept what they have been told. They are not the passive respondents to dominant forces, but actively disrupt received wisdoms, tactically subverting in everyday life dominant discourses (de Certeau 1984) to accommodate their own understandings, values and making things work for them. This presents a much more dynamic view of CAM use than the views underpinning efforts to identify particular reasons for CAM use discussed in the previous section. The healthcare journeys that people take are incredibly varied and unique, and the following provides illustrations of that variety.

Householders in this research were asked to draw a map of their house and indicate where medications were kept (Hodgetts et al. 2011). They were then asked to bring all the medications out that they would be happy to discuss and place them on the kitchen or coffee table, or the sitting room floor or wherever the discussion about medications was to take place. The medications, remedies and potions were then picked up, held in the hand of the householders and talked about. How did this medication get here? Who was it for and why? How did you decide to get this particular medication and so on? Many householders were shocked at what they saw in front of them once all the medications were recovered. They had no idea that they had stored so much in the house, in kitchen pantries, bathroom cabinets, bedside drawers and hallway cupboards – some hidden away and some proudly displayed.

Many households use what could be termed folk remedies. For example, household remedies used for 'sore throats and things' can engender a long list of responses, such as lemon, honey, ginger tea, salt and water. Recommended prescriptions from outside the household could be supplemented with others, such as antibiotics with self-prescribed probiotics or high doses of vitamin C. These everyday practices were also noted in the Indian subcontinent and in China in previous chapters and are likely to be evident across the globe.

Householders commonly deviate from the recommendations made by prescribers and others, whether orthodox or unorthodox, tactically engaging with them and adapting them to their own interests and rules (de Certeau 1984). Householders might outrightly reject medications prescribed by medical doctors, such as antibiotics, by drawing on their own understandings of what they might need to combat infection. Some householders would seek out alternatives to synthesised drugs prescribed by their doctor, so rather than using diuretics prescribed by her orthodox doctor, one householder stated 'It's better to just drink water and that flushes it through and have parsley tea and stuff – natural diuretics' (Dew et al. 2014).

Equally, householders could reject advice from alternative practitioners. Janice (all names used are pseudonyms) rejects a candidate diagnosis from an osteopath that she had scleroderma as she googled the term and found that she had 'less than five percent of the symptoms'. Ingrid takes a prescribed sleeping pill, but she does not tell her ayurvedic practitioner 'because he'd likely have a heart attack! He can't believe that somebody would have a problem with not sleeping'. In this instance, Ingrid is deviating from the recommendations of an alternative practitioner to follow more conventional advice. By contrast, Janice provides an account of having bowel problems and her doctor suggesting 'Basically don't eat anything that's going to stimulate your bowel and then just do it manually every day by using an enema'. Janice did not pursue this advice and instead followed the advice of her naturopath to take an appetite stimulant.

Some householders had developed a particular expertise in wellness practices. For example, Fleur had an expertise in homeopathic diagnosis and prescribing and all her family members took homeopathic medicines. She used different doses and prescribed for a wide range of conditions including infection, overeating and sunstroke, and her son stated, 'We even treat the dog'. Sylvia had developed expertise in the use of essential oils and some she would 'recommend to all and sundry', especially her four-year-old daughter and husband, but for some of the oils she would suggest that others should consult with a professional 'who knows them better than I do'. Here, households are sites of truth production, where through observation, research and experimentation treatment plans can be made, but limitations are placed around the application of their expertise. For some, their lack of expertise was a concern. Bryce notes that in the supermarket 'at least half of one side of an aisle is just medications' and, 'You can take all these things without actually knowing what they're doing to you or how they could interact with each other. All the adverse effects'.

Householders can become experts through their own training and through necessity, but also through processes of experimentation to determine such things as the right dose for them, when to take medications and when not to. Ingrid knew that if she took too much vitamin C 'it gives you diarrhoea. That's how you know so you don't do that'. Louisa was taking a homeopathic medication for urinary tract infection (UTI): 'I got to three drops once a day then I started having UTIs so I did four drops once a day. Hallelujah, it seemed to work so I left it at that'. Others go through a long process of experimentation that may go from homeopathic medicine to supplements to herbalism to Chinese medicine in efforts to find an approach that works for them. Someone else tries arnica for an ankle problem, then after reading on the topic considers acupuncture, then asks around to get a recommendation. This strategy evolves in dynamic fashion as different sources of information are drawn on. The dynamic unfolding of decision-making to use CAM problematises those efforts to find out some specific rationale for its use. A process of trial, error and retrial is common in households as they seek to redress unresolved health issues.

Some householders are well aware of the difficulties of determining causes from simple observation. Avril did not want to take antibiotic cream for rosacea, a skin condition that causes rashes on the face, so she tried 'a strange mixture of herbs'. Her condition improved but she stated:

> I don't know if it's the change of season but my rosacea is much less bad than it was. It was all lumpy and now it's gone smooth. So whether or not it was related to that Chinese herb I don't know.

Similarly, she stated that after taking a homeopathic remedy for hay fever, where she was 'sneezing really terribly' she subsequently:

> Didn't have any trouble for the rest of the day. Whether or not it was that or it was just coincidence but anyway, it seemed worth it for the sugar pill or whatever it is [laughter].

Coincidence and the idea of a sugar pill (a synonym for a placebo) are given some weight as possible explanations here. This ambivalence is further played out as Avril refers to another homeopathic remedy where she 'didn't notice any difference whatsoever'. So, Avril self-observes and notes changes but is cautious about assigning positive effects to the alternative medications she tries, though she is more emphatic in noting when they do not work. We can see Avril working to represent herself as someone who is not easily duped by the claims of others, but who can exercise scepticism appropriate to a scientifically informed person. The shadowy effects of the scientific methods and its stipulations causing people to question their own observation play out in everyday therapeutic activity. At the same time, people question the recommendations of experts, both orthodox and unorthodox, drawing on their own experiences, observations and determinations of therapeutic efficacy,

As noted, people have a wide range of sources of advice on therapeutic possibilities, with different hierarchies of trust and credibility. For some, chiropractors could be placed at the top of the hierarchy of trust and expertise for what is considered to be their knowledge of how systems work and interact. For others, what is trusted is an outcome of practicality and their own common sense. We can see this in one participant's explanation of why she took advice from her pharmacist about treatment for her heartburn. Her heartburn was a result of taking Nurofen for period pain. Her doctor had suggested taking an additional medication to 'mask the side effects of the acid', which Hazel thought was 'a very dumb thing to do'. Her nutritionist had 'more of an extreme view probably about diets and things like that and it would be a long-term approach – this really perfect diet all the time'. Instead of these 'extremes', she went to the pharmacist who advised omega oils, which for her was a middle way. This participant works through her health advisors until she obtains the advice that suited her.

Health professionals could also play a role in legitimating decisions. Zoe saw that her physiotherapist had Anti-Flamme in the consulting room, a herb-based medication, and because her physiotherapist used it that gave her confidence in its use. Zoe does not have so much faith in people who prescribe remedies. Relatives and friends are also sources of strategies. Hazel takes a zinc formula for colds recommended by her brother, and she also used grapefruit seed extract as she had had 'a few funny years of poor health'. She took it on the advice from a friend:

> She's a nurse, her husband's a doctor but they're also into alternative medicines themselves . . . If you look on the Internet, in fact, with this it's not clear. It doesn't have lots of research and there's actually websites that say, 'Don't take this stuff, it's toxic' . . . I do think what triggered it was my friend suggesting it.

Hazel here considers different sources of information before following the advice of a friend with high health cultural capital. Tania had a friend who is a naturopath and so is 'immersed in that world as well'. Avril and her partner 'know quite a few people who are into some kind of healing or another', including acupuncturists, osteopaths and chiropractors. Sylvia had endometriosis that conventional approaches had not resolved and a friend said 'look, I've heard this stuff's really good, why don't you go and have a chat to them?' referring to aromatherapy, to which Sylvia became a strong convert.

In a household with a tradition of using homeopathic remedies, we see a form of cultural or social capital at play around medication expertise, with the household drawing on strong family networks. The following relates to a hypothetical discussion about sore throats, where Jason, the son, just asks his mother for advice. Fleur, the mother, says 'we'd be giving them some echinacea straight away and then if it carried on then we might be going onto something else' and if required 'we'd be ringing up my mother [who is a homeopath] and, 'What do we need for this kind of symptom and that kind of symptom?'. In this instance, the mother claims a particular level of expertise, but calls on her own mother's expertise in situations that are not so common. Tania took psyllium hulls to promote bowel motions, as suggested by her mother, who was 'diagnosed with cancer thirty-eight years ago' and subsequently 'went totally holistic'. Orthodox prescriptions are also transferred across generations. Hazel takes Ibuprofen when menstrual pain stops her sleeping, something 'my Mum told me about'. Similarly, Sylvia used Bonjela teething gel for her baby, stating it was 'my Mum who told me about this'. In these data, men did not note intergenerational influences and fathers were not identified as important in health networks.

Workplaces act as a source of therapeutic information that comes into the household. Talk over lunchbreaks can introduce workmates to different therapeutic approaches, and colleagues might learn what others keep in their first aid kits or the drawers in their office desks, such as rescue remedy (a Bach flower remedy used to deal with stress and other conditions) or supplements. Colleagues may have special knowledge that can be passed on, attained through their own networks or even have training in some modality. Workplaces are then sources of information and spaces of observation and can provoke research into wellness strategies that are deployed in the home.

It is well established that people use the Internet to access information about medications (Nettleton 2004). The Internet can be used to access material from trusted sources and organisations, as with Sylvia who, in relation to the use of essential oils, states that 'there's a couple of very reputable international websites . . . you can soon find people who are actually trained who aren't going to put you wrong'. The Internet can be used to try and locate specific treatment advice. Avril used the Internet to explore orthodox options for her jaw clenching and noted that besides a splint 'they don't propose any alternatives'. This gave her licence to explore other options outside dentistry. Identifying wellness strategies could also be less systematic. Hazel took selenium because she 'read an article that really influenced me years ago about how there's very little selenium or none in the New Zealand soil'.

What we can learn from an examination of the therapeutic practices in households is that there is a great deal of activity that goes on here that could justify seeing households as therapeutic centres in their own right. Therapeutic approaches are sought out, used, assessed and adapted. Trusted regimes are called upon and new scenarios are responded to. What comes to dominate in practice will vary from household to household, and what combinations of practices are called upon will be unique to each household. The disciplinary processes of the state, the professions and forms of quality control and competency assessment discussed in Chapter 2 and 3 do not have such a strong hold inside the home. Therapeutic hybridity and blending abounds as statist medicine is reduced to one therapeutic approach amongst others.

CAM in the consultation

The hybrid nature of therapeutic practices in the home can contrast with how CAM is considered in the consultation (Dew 2016; Dew et al. 2008). In the following, the focus is on the unfolding of interactions when patients who are attending an orthodox practitioner consider heterodox options for their treatment.

The examples discussed occur in the context of audio- and video-recorded consultations in New Zealand. They come from a database of 105 patient consultations with nine GPs. In New Zealand, only one-third of patients who use CAM disclose this to their medical practitioner (Nicholson 2006). The New Zealand Health Practitioners Competence Assurance Act of 2003, which covers GPs and other medical practitioners, states that a practitioner cannot be found guilty of a disciplinary offence 'merely because that person has adopted and practised any theory of medicine or healing if, in doing so, the person has acted honestly and in good faith' (Medical Council of New Zealand 2005). The Medical Council of New Zealand's guidelines for medical practitioners who use CAM places the onus on the practitioners 'to inform the patient not only of the nature of the alternative treatment offered but also the extent to which that is consistent with conventional theories of medicine' (Medical Council of New Zealand 2005).

In the first example, taken from an interaction between a patient and a GP in a clinic, a patient makes a request for a blood test, but when queried about this, a problem arises when the patient suggests that he wants to follow an alternative diet. In this consultation, the clinician is looking at the computer and talking to the patient. The patient has explained what he wants the blood tests for by making reference to an unorthodox approach to dieting known as the blood type diet, which has been disparagingly referred to as a fad diet but one that gained popularity when followed by some famous actors. The premise of this diet is that the variety of food you eat should be based on your blood type, so for example, someone with blood type O should have a high protein diet whereas someone with A should have a diet based on fruit and vegetables. This is clearly an approach that does not align with orthodox nutritional and dietary advice. And this becomes quickly apparent in the consultation.

The unfolding of this interaction is as follows. The patient asks 'do you know what my blood type is' the GP says no but says a test can be done that has a small charge. The patient then goes on to explain why he wants the test, it is because he 'was thinking maybe doing a diet . . . it's good to know what your blood type is and they tell you what type of food to eat'. At this point, the GP stops looking at the computer and turns to the patient, she says 'oh yeah' and takes an in-breath, but before she says anything the patient has already realised he has transgressed and done something wrong, and he says 'or not'. The GP goes on to suggest that 'none of these diets have any great basis' and that 'the Mediterranean diet's we're all supposed to be eating'. The patient fulsomely agrees with this. From here on, the patient strongly affiliates with anything the clinician says in what appears to be an effort to change the topic as quickly as possible. The patient completely surrenders to the GP's perspective. In some consultations, like the one depicted in this scenario, we can see how attuned the patient is to 'illegitimate' knowledge, how quickly positions can change and how little evidence is required when one 'legitimate' view dominates. In this interaction, the doctor has worked to steer the patient away from something but has not explored why the patient was drawn to the diet in the first place, and this issue is not revisited in the consultation. The doctor's advice may or may not be taken up outside of the clinic. The patient may have retracted his request and interactionally aligned with the expert, but once outside it is possible he will pursue his interest in fad diets by other routes. As noted in the last section, patients may well pursue advice that aligns with their own understandings and values.

In another consultation, a patient refers to an interaction with what he describes as a 'health shop freak' who told the patient that his 'butt problems' could be a result of a medication he was using to reduce acid production in his stomach. The GPs immediate response to this piece of information is to align with the patient's description of someone as a freak, and he humorously says 'just tell him to naff off'. This seemingly knee-jerk reaction to someone countering the GPs advice is then revisited by the GP, who notes that he has 'wondered' about the impact of reducing acid in the stomach. Whilst the GP is pondering this issue the patient says he is not taking the medication anyway, and so signalling that he has aligned with the health shop freak, and the GP goes on to suggest that he would be 'very happy' to have the patient stop the medication (Dew et al. 2008). This interaction shows how people can come to their own decisions, weighing up advice from doctors and others and acting on their own assessment of that advice. The patient did not consult the GP about stopping medications but stopped taking the medications on the basis of his own understanding and response to alternative health advice he was given.

In some cases of CAM talk, the GP explicitly reserves judgement of CAM by withholding any response to the patient's talk. A woman consulting her GP about sores on her body tells the GP that she has been applying calendula cream, a homeopathic remedy used for skin irritation, and tea tree oil, an alternative antiseptic. These are not conventional medical approaches, but neither are they particularly challenging to orthodox medical practice in this consultation. The GP's response is neutral. She neither praises the patient for self-medicating using CAM approaches nor provides a negative response to the patient's story. She does not engage with the alternative approaches at all. Again, we see someone making their own decision without being given permission by experts from the dominant biomedical paradigm.

Rarely, a GP might suggest to a patient that she could use some alternative form of treatment, but this can be done with significant hedging, such as telling the patient that there is little proven about its efficacy, but the patient might feel better taking it. For example, in a consultation about premenstrual problems that are not responding to orthodox medicine, the GP suggests trialling evening primrose oil purchased from the chemist, or the chemist may have some other premenstrual preparation. The GP suggests that there is not the research to back it up but some people appear to be helped, but concludes that 'I wouldn't be surprised if things just settle down' (Dew et al. 2008). In this case, the GP suggests something alternative, without actively endorsing it. To endorse the product would not align with the New Zealand Medical Council guidelines on advising about CAM practices in this context. The doctor has signalled the lack of an evidence base for the option and in addition has qualified the chances of success of the treatment. The option works sometimes for some people, but will not necessarily work this time or for this patient. In this example, the dominant biomedical approach has failed, and so the GP tentatively indicates a non-orthodox direction that the patient might consider. Additionally, the GP places faith in the self-limiting nature of many conditions and that the problem may resolve without any intervention.

A contrasting example can be seen in the following extract drawn from a consultation with a patient for whom English is a second language and who has substituted a prescribed medication with a CAM medication. The patient tells the GP that she was taking a cholesterol lowering drug that the GP had prescribed to her, but she stopped using it as she couldn't sleep. So she went to the chemist who provided her with an alternative, and her sleep patterns returned to normal. The GP raises a concern about this unknown-to-her alternative prescription in that it might interact with other medications the patient is on, and so the GP suggests taking the cholesterol lowering medication at a different time of the day in the hope that it would prevent the insomnia.

The GP has to respond to the patient not only self-medicating but not complying and in addition to this, non-complying in a situation where the patient is on other medication. The GP does not question the possible efficacy of the CAM medication – 'it may well be that it works perfectly well' – but in this instance raises a concern about interactions with blood pressure medication. The GP states that she cannot guarantee that the substituted medication would not interact with the patient's other medications, which has the implication that the drug the GP prescribed would not interact with those other medications. The GP however goes to great lengths to preserve the patient's autonomy by framing the countermand as a tentative proposal, something that is a concern to the GP from her point of view, and that she would prefer it, and be happier, if the patient went back on to the prescribed medication. In an environment where patient rights are given some prominence, the GP negotiates a delicate balance between persuading the patient to do something that the GP thinks is in her best interests, but not making that a demand.

The following describes quite a different encounter, where a GP who also describes himself as a naturopath, offers the possibility of an alternative approach from a biomedical one. In doing so, he undertakes a great deal of interactional work, making the consultations longer and more complex than standard consultations. The following example is exceptional for the elaborate detail on the cause and treatment of the condition that is provided, but this is only after the GP has determined that the patient is open to the possibility of, in this instance, dietary change. The professional disciplinary environment in which this GP is working means it is important that he is not seen as imposing an approach on a patient that the patient might not want. For example, in a well-publicised case, a practitioner was de-registered in part as a result of being seen to impose his ideas on an unwilling patient (New Zealand Medical Journal 2004).

This is also a notable consultation in that the GP offers the patient a range of alternatives to the condition. In the data set that this consultation was drawn from (over 100 consultations recorded), it is not common for GPs to go into a detailed discussion of causation and physiological mechanisms, but rather, GPs proffer a diagnosis or possible diagnosis, and on occasion a brief explanation about causation. As such, GPs could be seen to draw on a common stock of knowledge that requires little in the way of elaboration. When this naturopathically influenced GP suggests dietary change, his explanation is very elaborate. In this consultation, a test has identified that the patient's cholesterol levels have risen. The GP has established that the patient does not know what the implications of this are and briefly outlines the risk for heart disease. The GP then provides an account of cholesterol and its functions, in far more detail than any other consultation about any other condition. There is no comparable discussion of physiology in the entire data set. The GP then moves on to discuss what can be done, suggesting that the patient has to weigh up the costs and benefits of the treatment options.

The GP makes it clear to the patient that he does not have to follow any suggested course of action, so avoiding any potential charge of coercion that might fall foul of Medical Council disciplinary procedures. The GP suggests that the options for the patient are to do nothing, to modify his diet and exercise, to take a pharmaceutical medication or to take a natural supplement. The patient responds by saying he favours the diet and exercise option. The GP then goes through a series of questions about current dietary practices with suggestions for change.

In doing so, the GP provides a detailed narrative outlining his theory of diet. He opens this with a preamble arguing that the modern diet has much lower protein consumption that the 'hunter gatherer' diet. The GP then goes on to say that the dietary advice provided by the government and the Ministry of Health is 'bunkum' and that they don't know what they are talking about. Following this very strong statement about the inadequacies of orthodox dietary advice, the narrative element is embarked upon where the GP relates contemporary dietary practices to the diet of Palaeolithic times, concluding by highlighting the importance of having protein at every meal. The patient expresses strong interest in this approach, saying it is a 'fantastic new picture for me' (Dew et al. 2008). The GP then suggests that he has a lot more to say but the consultation has been 'half an hour already and I've got people waiting'.

The GP has spent the equivalent of two appointment sessions describing to the patient the physiology of the 'problem' and his theory of causation and treatment, and addressing specific dietary changes that the patient can make. It is likely that this relates to the GP's particular consultation style, although his other consultations where orthodox treatments are discussed are nothing like as comprehensive as this one. It does raise the possibility that for some GPs CAM issues are more time consuming. Johanna Ruusovuori (2007) makes a somewhat similar observation in her analysis of Finnish homeopathic consultations. The data are also suggestive of the lengths to which GPs who recommend alternative approaches can go to present an alternative explanation of disease and its treatment. This points to an extra burden that GPs who uses CAM may have to carry, that is, more interactional work and potentially longer consultations.

From observing these consultations, we can note that patients initiate talk about CAM in diverse contexts that raise different issues for GPs. In the research discussed here, when individual CAM practitioners are mentioned by the patients, the GP responses are not positive and in some instances are overtly negative. However, it should not be assumed that this demonstrates that GPs have negative views of CAM as the GPs may be involved in relational work when they do this. That is, GPs commonly have continuity of care with patients and they would be unlikely to unnecessarily challenge a patient on views unless they were of clinical importance. However, while the orthodox GPs' responses to CAM are often cautious and while they might criticise individual CAM practitioners, they are nevertheless careful in when and how they are dismissive of CAM itself. If possible, they align with any negative appraisal of CAM by the patient, but in a sense give permission to adopt CAM if it does not compromise an orthodox approach. For this reason, supplementation per se elicits neutral responses from the GPs but substitution elicits a negative response. It may be the case that a boundary issue between acceptable and unacceptable CAM practices can be identified here – where substitution by patients intrudes overtly on the medical domain and therefore is rejected.

One clear transgression is where a patient has substituted a CAM option for a prescribed medication. Another potential transgression issue is where patients take advice from CAM practitioners or advocates. In other words, CAM practices are not negatively judged in themselves by GPs unless they transgress on their medical prescribing or where the role of GPs as advisors is directly challenged. In addition, CAM practitioners themselves who provide alternative advice and diagnoses are liable to intrude on the GP's domain. However, any rejection of CAM is carefully crafted by the GP, so as not to challenge or threaten patients in relation to their choices. Not surprisingly then, we see the biomedical paradigm being asserted in these consultations, but there is room around the edges to accommodate some limited use of CAM. As a caveat, there will be a much greater diversity of responses to CAM in the consultation than considered here. The consultations discussed took place in New Zealand on a self-selecting sample of GPs who were enabling the research to be undertaken on aspects of health communication. Even within these limitations, a sense of the constraints on GPs can be discerned.

The variety of responses seen in this data set is in line with other research looking at patients and practitioners in relation to CAM. Philip Tovey and Alex

Broom (2007) note that oncology patients report three types of approach to CAM from oncologists – explicit or implicit negativity, supportive ambivalence and pragmatic acceptance. Supportive ambivalence is where the oncologists were not supportive of CAM but were supportive of patient choice, and pragmatic acceptance describes situations where oncologists would actively support patients' use of CAM and even refer patients to CAM practitioners. Different GP relationships to CAM can be delineated, including CAM approaches as ones to be rejected even if there is little else to offer from a biomedical perspective, CAM approaches as complementary, so that they can be added to orthodox approaches and might work, and CAM approaches as radical alternatives based on a different understanding to conventional medical theories.

Concluding comments

The term habitus, as developed by Pierre Bourdieu, has usefully been deployed to provide insight into the way people decide on therapeutic choices and negotiate pathways through them (Hansen et al. 2020 (early online)). Habitus refers to a socialised or structured body that shapes perception and action in the world, captured in the view that 'w]hile individuals choose their lifestyle they are, however, predisposed by their habitus toward certain choices' (Frohlich et al. 2001).

In this chapter, I have provided an overview of different views on why people use CAM. There is no simple answer to this. Reasons are diverse, with the experience of chronic conditions not satisfactorily treated by biomedicine prominent. The concept of habitus can go some way in explaining different kinds of responses that people take. But when we look at how people make decisions and how they practice therapeutics in the home, the contingent nature of CAM use comes to the fore. Certainly, therapeutic practices and responses to illness can be passed down through the generations, and people respond to dominant understandings, but they also come across articles, hear talk and experiment with possibilities. It is at this level, the individual embedded in their networks of connections that therapeutic possibilities operate as a kaleidoscopic spectacle. Therapeutic pluralism does not capture the ways in which people mix and match, blend or integrate different therapeutic approaches. A hybrid therapeutics is in operation.

Back in the consultation rooms, we see a delicate and intricate dance, as the therapeutic hybridity meets biomedical dominance. But this dominance is not hegemonic for everyone. The biomedical has to accommodate a more empowered patient. In this space, we also see the even more delicate balance and dance of the unorthodox GP, who has to operate in a way that is less economically efficient than his more orthodox colleagues, and has to make therapeutic recommendations in ways that avoids the possibility of disciplinary action coming from his profession.

Globally, at the level of the consumer, patient, healthcare user and householder, the shifting and dynamic terrain of therapeutic possibilities is most clearly manifested.

References

Arnold, D. (2018) Technology and health in late colonial India, in R.D. Roy and G.N.A. Attewell (eds.), *Locating the medical*, Oxford: Oxford University Press, pp. 264–284.

Baarts, C. and Pedersen, I.K. (2009) Derivative benefits: Exploring the body through complementary and alternative medicine, *Sociology of Health & Illness*, 31, 5, 719–733.

Barnes, P., Bloom, B. and Nahin, R. (2008) Complementary and alternative medicine use among adults and children: United States, 2007, *National Health Statistics Reports*, 10, 12, 1–23.

Chamberlain, K., Madden, H., Gabe, J., Dew, K. and Norris, P. (2011) Forms of resistance to medication within New Zealand households, *Medische Anthroplogie*, 23, 2, 299–308.

Clavarino, A. and Yates, P. (1995) Fear, faith or rational choice: Understanding the users of alternative therapies, in G. Lupton and J. Najman (eds.), *Sociology of health and illness: Australian readings*, Melbourne: Macmillan, pp. 252–275.

Consumers' Institute (1997) Non-conventional therapies: From arsenic to zinc, *Consumer*, 363, 20–27.

Coward, R. (1989) *The whole truth: The myth of alternative health*, London: Faber.

de Certeau, M. (1984) *The practice of everyday life*, Berkeley: University of California Press.

Dew, K. (2016) Purifying and hybridising categories in healthcare decision-making: The clinic, the home and the multidisciplinary team, *Health Sociology Review*, 25, 2, 142–156.

Dew, K., Chamberlain, K., Hodgetts, D., Norris, P., Radley, A. and Gabe, J. (2014) Home as a hybrid centre of medication practice, *Sociology of Health & Illness*, 36, 1, 28–43.

Dew, K., Norris, P., Gabe, J., Chamberlain, K. and Hodgetts, D. (2015) Moral discourses and pharmaceuticalised governance in households, *Social Science & Medicine*, 131, 272–279.

Dew, K., Plumridge, E., Stubbe, M., Dowell, A., Macdonald, L. and Major, G. (2008) 'You just got to eat healthy': The topic of CAM in the general practice consultation, *Health Sociology Review*, 17, 4, 396–409.

Frank, R. and Stollberg, G. (2004) Medical acupuncture in Germany: Patterns of consumerism among physicians and patients, *Sociology of Health & Illness*, 26, 3, 351–372.

Frohlich, K.L., Corin, E. and Potvin, L. (2001) A theoretical proposal for the relationship between context and disease, *Sociology of Health & Illness*, 23, 6, 776–797.

Hansen, F., Berntsen, G.R. and Salamonsen, A. (2020, early online) Medical pluralism in the aftermath of cancer health seeking actions and cancer patients' shaping of trajectories to healing, *Anthropology & Medicine*, 1–17.

Harris, P. and Rees, R. (2000) The prevalence of complementary and alternative medicine use among the general population: A systematic review of the literature, *Complementary Therapies in Medicine*, 8, 2, 88–96.

Hess, D.J. (2004) Medical modernisation, scientific research fields and the epistemic politics of health social movements, *Sociology of Health & Illness*, 26, 6, 695–709.

Hodgetts, D., Chamberlain, K., Gabe, J., Dew, K., Radley, A., Madden, H., Norris, P. and Waimarie Nikora, L. (2011) Emplacement and everyday use of medications in domestic dwellings, *Health & Place*, 17, 1, 353–360.

Hodgetts, D., Young-Hauser, A., Chamberlain, K., Gabe, J., Dew, K. and Norris, P. (2017) Pharmaceuticalisation in the city, *Urban Studies*, 54, 15, 3542–3559.

Jakes, D. and Kirk, R. (2015) How and why patients use acupuncture: An interpretive phenomenological study, *Journal of Primary Health Care*, 7, 2, 124–129.

Kelner, M. and Wellman, B. (1997) Health care and consumer choice: Medical and alternative therapies, *Social Science & Medicine*, 45, 2, 203–212.

Latour, B. (1993) *We have never been modern*, Cambridge, MA: Harvard University Press.

Lynöe, N. and Svensson, T. (1992) Physicians and alternative medicine: An investigation of attitudes and practice, *Scandinavian Journal of Social Medicine*, 20, 1, 55–60.

Marshall, R.J. and Gee, R. (1990) The use of alternative therapies by Auckland general practitioners, *New Zealand Medical Journal*, 103, 889, 213–215.

Medical Council of New Zealand (2005) *Statement on complementary and alternative medicine*, Wellington: Medical Council of New Zealand.

Murray, J. and Shepherd, S. (1993) Alternative or additional medicine? An exploratory study in general practice, *Social Science & Medicine (1982)*, 37, 8, 983.

Nettleton, S. (2004) The emergence of e-scaped medicine?, *Sociology*, 38, 4, 661–679.

New Zealand Medical Journal (2004) Medical discipline: Alternative medicine, *New Zealand Medical Journal*, 117, 1191.

Nicholls, P. (1988) *Homoeopathy and the medical profession*, London: Croom Helm.

Nicholson, T. (2006) Complementary and alternative medicines (including traditional Māori treatments) used by presenters to an emergency department in New Zealand: A survey of prevalence and toxicity, *New Zealand Medical Journal*, 119, 1233.

Northcott, H. and Bachynsky, J. (1993) Concurrent utilization of chiropractic, prescription medicines, nonprescription medicine and alternative health care, *Social Science & Medicine*, 37, 3, 431–435.

Parliament of Victoria Social Development Committee (1986) *Inquiry into alternative medicine and the health food industry*, Melbourne: Parliament of Victoria.

Parsons, T. (1958) Definitions of health and illness in the light of American values, in E.G. Jaco (ed.), *Patients, physicians and illness: Sourcebook in behavioral science and medicine*, Glencoe: The Free Press, pp. 165–187.

Penney, L.S., Ritenbaugh, C., Elder, C., Schneider, J., Deyo, R.A. and Debar, L.L. (2016) Primary care physicians, acupuncture and chiropractic clinicians, and chronic pain patients: A qualitative analysis of communication and care coordination patterns, *BMC Complementary and Alternative Medicine*, 16, 29, 30.

Possamai-Inesedy, A. and Cochrane, S. (2013) The consequences of integrating complementary and alternative medicine: An analysis of impacts on practice, *Health Sociology Review*, 22, 1, 65–74.

Ruusovuori, J. (2007) Managing affect: The integration of empathy and problem-solving in health care encounters, *Discourse Studies*, 9, 5, 597–622.

Saks, M. (2001) Alternative medicine and the health care division of labour: Present trends and future prospects, *Current Sociology*, 49, 3, 119–134.

Sharma, U. (1992) *Complementary medicine today: Practitioners and patients*, London: Routledge.

——— (1996) Using complementary therapies: A challenge to orthodox medicine?, in S.J. Williams and M. Calnan (eds.), *Modern medicine: Lay perspectives and experiences*, London: UCL Press, pp. 230–255.

Sharp, D., Lorenc, A., Little, P., Mercer, S.W., Hollinghurst, S., Feder, G. and MacPherson, H. (2018) Complementary medicine and the NHS: Experiences of integration with UK primary care, *European Journal of Integrative Medicine*, 24, 8–16.

Siahpush, M. (1998) Postmodern values, dissatisfaction with conventional medicine and popularity of alternative therapies, *Journal of Sociology*, 34, 58–70.

Sointu, E. (2006) The search for wellbeing in alternative and complementary health practices, *Sociology of Health & Illness*, 28, 330–349.

——— (2012) *Theorizing complementary and alternative medicines: Wellbeing, self, gender, class*, Basingstoke: Palgrave.

Steel, A., Frawley, J., Adams, J., Sibbritt, D. and Broom, A. (2013) Primary health care, complementary and alternative medicine and women's health: A focus upon menopause, in J. Adams, P. Magin and A. Broom (eds.), *Primary health care and complementary and integrative medicine: Practice and research*, London: Imperial College Press, pp. 11–33.

Tovey, P. and Broom, A. (2007) Oncologists' and specialist cancer nurses' approaches to complementary and alternative medicine and their impact on patient action, *Social Science & Medicine*, 64, 12, 2550–2564.

Willison, K., Lindsay, S., Taylor, M., Schroeder, H. and Andrews, G. (2013) Complementary and integrative medicine, aging and chronic illness: Towards an interprofessional approach in primary health care, in J. Adams, P. Magin and A. Broom (eds.), *Primary health care and complementary and integrative medicine: Practice and research*, London: Imperial College Press, pp. 35–49.

Xue, C.C.L., Zhang, A.L., Lin, V., Da Costa, C. and Story, D.F. (2007) Complementary and alternative medicine in Australia: A national population-based survey, *Journal of Alternative and Complementary Medicine*, 13, 6, 643–650.

8

THE FRAUGHT USE OF CAM IN CANCER CARE

Cancer is a disease that, when diagnosed, is likely to evoke fear and dread. It is, furthermore, a site of extremes of treatment. For many cancers, a conventional medical approach is chemotherapy, the use of highly toxic drugs to try to eliminate any traces of cancer. Other treatments can be equally as taxing, such as radiotherapy and surgery. It can only be expected that in the face of such toxic and at times debilitating treatments, which have variable success rates, many would turn to alternative approaches.

This chapter will consider how and why people use CAM, the use of CAM practices in biomedical cancer care settings and the understandings of CAM practitioners about cancer causation and treatment. The use of medicinal cannabis for the treatment of cancer and other conditions will be considered as it provides intriguing insights into the relationships around statist medicine and subaltern therapeutic practices around the charged issue of cancer care.

Many people diagnosed with cancer will use CAM, usually alongside biomedical interventions. The rates of CAM use by people diagnosed with cancer vary a great deal across countries, types of cancer and also particular population groups under study, with the low end of the range for use around one-third of patients and the higher end approaching ninety percent (Molassiotis et al. 2005). Some of the high end of the range for CAM use should be treated with caution. Cleora Roberts and colleagues' (2006) study of CAM use by cancer patients in the United States found that eighty-seven percent used CAM, but their definition includes exercise and prayer as complementary therapies. Patients with poor prognoses in conventional terms were the highest users of CAM (Molassiotis et al. 2005). As one of Rebecca Olson's participants stated, drawing on a complementary approach to Western medicine in the face of a poor prognosis for neurological cancer was done on the 'off chance' that it would help (Olson 2015).

The most popular therapies used tend to be dietary changes (including non-traditional or unorthodox diets), herbalism, homeopathy, hypnotherapy and visualisation approaches (Molassiotis et al. 2005). For many cancer patients who use CAM, the goal is not necessarily to treat the disease, but maybe to help with side effects and improve emotional well-being. Cancer patients can use CAM therapies to deal with the on-going consequences of the effects of the disease, diagnosis and treatment, such as dealing with the anxiety of relapse, existential questions that may be confronted when facing possible death or responding to physical issues like fatigue (Hansen et al. 2020). However, it is evident that in many situations we could anticipate that many cancer patients use CAM in some form.

By far, the majority of cancer patients who used CAM believed it was effective. Certain CAM approaches have gained some legitimacy through standardised trials, such as the use of acupuncture to help reduce the nausea that can follow chemotherapy, and the use of meditation approaches to reduce anxiety (Broom 2006). Many people used CAM before a diagnosis of cancer but post-diagnosis the rate of use increased (Molassiotis et al. 2005). Some patients used types of CAM they had not used before. For some CAM therapies, there was a drop-off in use following the diagnosis.

People who have prior investment in, or even a strong commitment to, CAM approaches in everyday healthcare practices might go in the opposite direction in the face of a cancer diagnosis. In research on household use of medications, one participant stated that she preferred naturopathic products to treat problems, but 'I suppose if I got cancer I would go straight to the allopathic stuff' (Chamberlain et al. 2011: 304). Thus, householders may draw on different forms of governance depending upon the situation.

One modality where there was a drop-off in use following a diagnosis of cancer was osteopathy (Molassiotis et al. 2005). My own training as an osteopath provides possible explanations for why osteopathy was singled out as a CAM therapy that dropped in use following a cancer diagnosis. One concern that was raised during my training was that the rhythmic movements of the body that some osteopaths used may have the effect of enhancing the flow of lymph, and that cancer can metastasise via the lymphatic system. Therefore, for some osteopaths, there might be a concern that their treatment ran the danger of facilitating metastases. Another concern was that if there is cancer in the bone then any efforts at directing physical force to the bones runs the danger of damaging the bones, so manipulation might be something to be avoided.

The relatively high use of CAM by cancer patients does have implications beyond the patient. For example, concerns have been raised about pharmaceutical trials on cancer patients, many of whom might be using CAM (Molassiotis et al. 2005). In one study, nearly two-thirds of patients in a cancer trial were using CAM (Roberts et al. 2006).

CAM in cancer care settings

Although many cancer patients use CAM, the majority of patients who do so do not inform their physicians of such use (Roberts et al. 2006). The reasons given by patients includes that their doctor did not ask and that they did not think it was relevant (Roberts et al. 2006). Not surprisingly then, physicians underestimate how many of their patients are using CAM, and oncology physicians are unlikely to raise the topic of CAM with their patients. In a US study, nine percent of doctors caring for cancer patients were very uncomfortable talking about the subject, and nearly eight percent had refused to provide treatment to patients because they were using unconventional treatments as well (Roberts et al. 2006). Although there are many more physicians who are comfortable talking about CAM, the impact of those who are not or who refuse treatment to those who use CAM may be considerable. From a biomedical perspective, this lack of knowledge about patient CAM use raises concern about potential interactions between CAM treatments, especially if they are remedy based, and biomedical treatment. For example, concerns have been raised that some ingested CAM products, such as fish oils and feverfew, may exacerbate surgical bleeding (Roberts et al. 2006).

Cancer consultations where CAM is made a topic can have untoward outcomes, and we can see how 'alternatives' come into being. This suggests that we should be cautious about considering biomedical approaches and alternatives as pregiven. They can become manifest, or be constructed, through interactions between people in the here and now. In the following example, taken from research with patients who had been diagnosed with cancer, the patient recalls a consultation where a treatment plan was being made in response to a cancer diagnosis (Dew et al. 2015a). The consultation was between a Māori patient and a non-Māori health practitioner. Māori are the indigenous people of New Zealand, and Māori may draw on therapeutic approaches that have been developed within Māori culture. The following transcript refers to rongoā, which is a Māori therapeutic approach to healing that can include spiritual healing, plant-based medicines and massage. In this excerpt from an interview with the patient, she provides an account of her response to suggestions made by the oncologist to have orthodox treatments for the cancer:

> I said, 'No, I'm not going that way. I'm going to stay with the rongoā'. The Māori herbal way. Because it was a holistic approach. And it clashed straight away . . . I walked out of that meeting. I ran out . . . I basically said, 'Get fucked to you,' and left . . . Because I didn't like . . . the fact that he could sit there and pooh pooh . . . my way of wanting to get it fixed at that time. And basically telling me I'm a dead person if I go the rongoā way.
>
> *Dew et al. (2015a: 146)*

In this instance, we see a very strong clash between different 'purified' approaches, one described as holistic by the interviewee, which is contrasted to whatever treatment she was being offered in the consultation with the oncologist. The woman perceived that the oncologist was ridiculing her approach. It is likely that the oncologist was trying to do what he thought was best for his patient, that she follows his prescribed pathway for a potentially life-threatening condition, a pathway which would have included very toxic and powerful chemotherapy drugs and perhaps radiotherapy. For this oncologist, there does not appear to be a way to integrate his patient's desire with his own goals. So, in this case, instead of an integrated approach or approaches that complement each other, exclusive alternatives are created. The categories of biomedicine and rongoā medicine stay separate and unconnected. This type of interaction may have several negative consequences. From a biomedical perspective, the patient may not access the desired treatment. From a healthcare perspective, the patient may have lost faith or trust in biomedicine and limit consultations with health professionals in the future. From a health intervention perspective, the patient may not have the opportunity to now use biomedical approaches.

Alternatives to this scenario can be envisaged. The participants could have constructed the two systems as complementary or as part of a continuum of treatment. The oncologist could have suggested trying the rongoā but having the patient's condition monitored, so that the option of more aggressive biomedical treatments could still be on the table.

In this instance, the patient had been to a Māori healer who said she would help her, but that her condition looked like cancer so she should have it checked out by her 'Pākehā [non- Māori] doctor'. The patient 'didn't trust the Western medical system' because in her view it belittled Māori medicine. She stated in relation to orthodox medical approaches that:

> Māori patients who've gone that way have died, and I tried to tell him a lot of Pākehā patients that have gone that way have died too . . . in fact I thought more people have died under the knife than under the holistic approach. So I just thought he had the cheek . . . it has never left my memory.
>
> *(cited in Dew et al. 2015a: 146)*

Here, we have a situation where relationships between the patient and her health professional have broken down because of a sense that the patient's approach is being belittled. The patient's resistance could of course have major consequences for her. The stakes may be very high, they may be life or death, they may include being alienated or comforted by the chosen therapeutic approach, and in this emotionally intense atmosphere, it may be unsurprising that antagonisms between different therapeutic approaches are also intensified.

In this research on cancer patients' journeys through New Zealand healthcare systems, we also witness contrasting situations. For example, in a case that seemed particularly difficult, the cancer health professional was quite happy for the patient to pursue an alternative approach (Dew et al. 2019). Moana (a pseudonym) is attending a radiation oncology consultation. She has chronic obstructive pulmonary disease and severely reduced activities. Any treatment related to a likely lung tumour is unlikely to be helpful and may cause further damage to the lungs. But Moana must make a decision about whether to go with some treatment that might have a small chance of helping or give up on treatment altogether. Moana makes a decision (quite rare in cancer care consultations, where many 'decisions' are more like informing patients of a treatment plan) to try out an alternative approach: 'apricot kernels, seeds . . . vitamins and all that sort of thing'. She states that by the next appointment 'I will have done a course of it, and we'll see where we are'. The oncologist does not challenge this decision, even though from a conventional perspective it would not be viewed as an effective approach and would be considered a waste of time and effort (as also seems to be the case with biomedical treatment in this situation). The oncologist allows this course of action in the face of biomedical approaches having nothing of substance to offer (Dew et al. 2019). In this context, treatment offered by the oncologist would be publicly funded, but none was clearly on offer. The patient, in an intolerable situation, was given license to pursue privately funded alternatives and therapeutic approaches that are unorthodox and generally frowned upon by biomedical practitioners.

Opting for alternative approaches in cancer care can lead to extraordinary stand-offs between patients or their families and medical professionals. An example of this is the Liam Williams-Holloway case that occurred in New Zealand during 1999 and 2000. In this case, medical practitioners were pitted against a family over the treatment of a child with cancer. The family went into hiding so that they could provide alternative treatment for their child, and the medical oncologists took legal action to make Liam a ward of court so that he could be compelled to receive orthodox treatment (Broom 2000). This case polarised public opinion on the use of alternative therapies for cancer, with some suggesting that it is a family's right to seek out the treatment they believe is best for their child, and others suggesting that designated experts should decide what is best.

There are situations, however, where CAM therapies can be used within biomedical settings. Oncologists tend to be supportive of patients using some forms of CAM, such as meditation and, if we conceptualise the following as CAM as Cleora Roberts and colleagues appear to, attending support groups and undertaking exercise (Roberts et al. 2006). In the United Kingdom, CAM modalities have been used inside hospitals to treat cancer patients and also in hospices. In a study by Alex Broom and Philip Tovey (2007), a hospital and a hospice in the United Kingdom offered a range of therapies, including aromatherapy massage, hypnotherapy, spiritual healing and reflexology, with all the CAM therapists providing their services free to cancer patients. Their reception by medical practitioners and their integration are quite different in these two spaces, but in both spaces modalities that challenged biomedical epistemologies, such as homeopathy and herbalism, were not offered. Arguably medical practitioners in this study were receptive to modalities that could be considered complementary but not receptive to ones that are alternative. A very constrained form of therapeutic pluralism operates.

Hospital oncology has a focus on disease whereas in hospices there is more of a focus on overall patient well-being (Broom and Tovey 2007). Hospices are not places of cure, but of comfort and care for the terminally ill. So, in the former the ideal of evidence-based assessments to gain legitimacy may prevail, whereas in the latter more subjective measures, such as patient satisfaction, may be more prominent. Despite many oncology treatments not being backed up by RCTs and being justified on the basis of clinical experience rather than the gold standard of biomedical evidence, medical oncologists will claim that CAM needs to have an evidence base before being supported (Broom and Tovey 2007) or at least the therapists must deploy a 'biomedically justifiable logic' (Broom and Tovey 2007: 558). That is, medical oncologists can entertain a shift from justifying a practice on the basis of evidence to a willingness to use evidence if it is available, but the evidence is that promoted by the evidence-based medicine movement. Broom and Tovey found that medical oncologists did not think CAM practitioners had that willingness and therefore those practitioners and their modalities should not be supported by funding (hence free services were OK) and referrals should not be made to CAM therapists. In the hospital setting, professional distance between CAM practitioners and medical practitioners was then maintained. Similar to many CAM therapies in oncology, there are few palliative care interventions that have attained the evidence-based threshold of RCTs. Palliative care practitioners then draw on their own observations and weaker forms of evidence to justify their practices.

The integration of CAM treatments into the institutions of biomedical care is an issue of some ambiguity for patients as well. In research on cancer patients who used CAM in the United Kingdom, it was found that patients were happy making their own decision about the benefits and costs of CAM, but were unclear about whether the NHS should provide CAM services as part of its cancer care services (Tovey and Broom 2008). Patient were aware of the power of existing bureaucracies in determining need and that public services worked within constrained budgets, and for many CAM services, they were not likely to meet the threshold of funding support. However, when it came to palliative care, there was much greater support for the use of CAM in hospices to attend to the different needs of the terminally ill. These CAM services were more of the variety to support emotional and spiritual needs rather than physical needs (Tovey and Broom 2008).

Patients who use CAM can be categorised in particular ways by cancer care health professionals. This can be seen in observations of cancer care multidisciplinary meetings in hospitals. Multidisciplinary meetings are team or group meetings with a wide range of clinicians and diagnosticians, which can include oncologists, pathologists, radiologists, oncology nurses and social workers. In a study of multidisciplinary meetings, I and my colleagues found that there was a fairly structured way of introducing cases (Dew et al. 2015b). In the introductions, age and gender were noted, and then a brief history of the case including investigations and treatments was conveyed. Very rarely were other categories used in the introduction, so when they were used, they seemed to be doing some sort of action. Occupation of the patient was one of these rarely mentioned categories. In one multidisciplinary meeting, the occupation of the patient was made relevant and she was described as a 'colour therapist'. The presenting clinician stated, 'My guess is that she will decline the offer of surgery'. The occupational category here implicitly linked to category bound activities like pursuing alternative treatments. Making occupation relevant thus supported the clinician's 'guess' that she might decline the suggested intervention (Dew et al. 2015b). This example alerts us to the ways in which people interact with others on the basis of how they categorise or classify each other. These categorisations do have consequences. To be classed as a CAM therapist in this case may influence the type of interaction that is had, maybe what services are offered and how strongly or not recommendations are made. We are all attuned to the power of these classifications, perhaps another reason why people are cautious about telling their health practitioners that they are using CAM, as that may have consequences for how they are classified.

Broom suggests that biomedicine strategically evolves in relation to CAM, basing this on evidence of medical oncologists claiming that they have a greater emphasis on patient well-being and encourage the use of relaxation techniques or other 'benign' CAM therapies like reiki. CAM therapists treating cancer patients may also strategically draw on biomedical approaches, such as herbalists pushing to use biomedical approaches to test effectiveness to support the use of their treatments (Broom 2006). Broom argues that, drawing on the work of Bruno Latour, we can fruitfully see this as a process of reciprocal inscription, where different approaches absorb elements from each other, rather than operate as binary opposites (Broom 2006). Arguably, reciprocal inscription operates at the margins of interactions between CAM and biomedicine in cancer care.

CAM users and cancer care

The use of CAM in the face of cancer has been seen to have a number of positive aspects, such as providing a sense of empowerment and control for patients and promoting hope. Many people combine chemotherapy and other aggressive medical approaches with meditation practices, mindfulness and mental imaging, and these practices have been associated with longer than expected survival (Cunningham et al. 2000). Research on exceptional cancer survivors found that in addition to conventional approaches, patients used a variety of CAM approaches, which Johanna Hök and colleagues (2009) classified as energy-based therapies, biologically based therapies, manipulative therapies and body-based therapies. Exceptional cancer survivors are deemed in this research to be people who have lived longer than expected. Hök and colleagues found that both biomedical health practitioners and alternative healing practitioners attributed patient survival with cancer to their own interventions; however, the patients who saw both, attributed survival to combinations of conventional and alternative treatments and their own actions and decisions, or agency. It seems that everyone involved believed in their own agency to effect change.

In the home, people can draw on a variety of evidence or sources. For instance, in research on householders' use of medications, discussed in Chapter 7, Paula has taken fish oil since she had breast cancer nineteen years ago: 'Whether it's done me any good I don't know but they tell me that nineteen years is a pretty good record for a person with breast cancer'. She thought 'that's probably mind over matter as well but I still take it . . . I mean, if people believe in it enough maybe that's part of the way of, you know, fixing it'. Paula is not taking fish oil because it was prescribed by a doctor but because she read an article by a naturopath 'that fish oil is very good for people that have breast cancer'. She has no clear evidence of it working, but she has come to trust in the restorative power of fish oil. Even if the oil itself is not therapeutic, for Paula, the belief itself is therapeutic (Dew 2018: 50).

Any therapeutic regimen requires forms of self-governance and using CAM brings into play particular forms of self-governance. Cancer survival strategies for those post-diagnosis are entwined with imperatives to diet, exercise and to have a positive mindset to prevent recurrence and progression of disease (Bell 2010). Some negative effects of such imperatives are seen in the use of CAM in cases of incurable cancer (Broom and Tovey 2008). In some situations, the use of alternative approaches can be at great personal and financial cost. Broom and Tovey highlight one case of a man in his eighties who undertakes a very rigorous and costly dietary regimen and the use of enemas to detoxify his body in an unsuccessful effort to keep the cancer at bay. The demands to take responsibility, and in this case to put so much energy into what was a futile attempt to extend life, takes its toll on individuals and their families. In Olson's study of caregivers of cancer patients, she found that for some patients with a terminal diagnosis using CAM allowed for a future focus and a greater sense of control with the hope of beating the cancer. In doing so, caregivers of cancer patients may spend hours in the kitchen preparing foods and spend thousands of dollars on remedies.

In contrast, Frank Hansen and colleagues discuss the case of Julie who initially wanted to respond to her colorectal cancer diagnosis by postponing conventional chemotherapy and radiation therapy until after she had tried alternative approaches, including the use of herbal preparations from India. However, she was convinced by her doctors not to postpone treatment. Her tumour shrank with treatment, which she put down to the herbal medicine she was using rather than the conventional treatment, but the latter had left her in chronic pain as the radiation therapy had harmed her bone structure. Julie regretted having gone down the conventional treatment pathway (Hansen et al. 2020).

The relationship between CAM, biomedicine and cancer varies hugely around the globe. In India, for example, much of the population do not have access to biomedical cancer care facilities and for those that do there is a strong gender bias. The cost of accessing biomedical care in a strongly patriarchal society can have the consequence that women and girl children are far less likely to receive biomedical care, and therefore, they are more reliant on cheaper alternative approaches that might be found in traditional practices such as ayurveda

(Broom et al. 2009). Oncologists and others providing therapeutic assistance to cancer patients may advise their patients to avoid using traditional therapies in their cancer treatment, but the physicians themselves may use these same therapeutic approaches in their own homes on an everyday basis (Broom et al. 2009). This alerts us to many issues. The structured nature and gendered bias are evident in India and we can observe other structural shapings in the West, such as the imperative to make efforts to extend one's life and live positively when responding to a cancer diagnosis. We also see differences between medical practitioners, such as oncologists as purveyors of a dominant ideology, and these same people, when needing therapeutic help, taking a pragmatic experimental approach to treatment. We also see diverse ways in which outcomes of interventions are assessed, with practitioners and patients having different understandings of treatment effects.

CAM practitioners

How CAM practitioners view cancer and its treatment can be gleaned from a US study of forty-six CAM practitioners involved in cancer care. The practitioners used a total of seventy different modalities and a great diversity of aetiologies for breast cancer were noted by the practitioners (Sered and Agigian 2008). Explanations provided for why a patient got breast cancer were external to the patient (for example, social and environmental issues) and internal, or based on the patient's own attitudes and decision-making, such as eating the wrong foods or having negative views. Practitioners usually did not have a notion of a single cause but of the body and mind being the subject of many damaging effects. Environmental concerns could be as broadly based as the notion of the earth itself being less pure, to concerns about pesticides, toxins like antibiotics in the food and generally vitiated foods. Social causes included excessive work and stressful work environments, individualised lifestyles with a lack of community connection and a lack of connection to the natural world.

Individual factors considered by CAM practitioners in the US study included the role of genetics, trauma that the patient had experienced before the onset of the cancer, which could be psychological trauma, particular character traits like a lack of self-esteem or the holding on to negative beliefs. These traits could be shaped by the gendered environment such as women tending to the needs of others and not their own or women being oppressed and not able to speak for themselves (Sered and Agigian 2008).

Susan Sered and Amy Agigian, the authors of this US study, use the concept of holistic sickening to capture the complex and interacting processes that are thought by the CAM practitioners to be the cause of cancer. They argue that their research aligns with the views of other scholars who see CAM as placing 'enormous emphasis upon the individual's responsibility for illness and little emphasis upon social-structural and environmental factors' (Sered and Agigian 2008: 627). Given the summary of their findings in the previous two paragraphs, this conclusion may seem peculiar, as the practitioners point to an array of factors and appear to provide a strong emphasis on the structured nature of cancer causation. But perhaps the difference here is between identifying a cause, that in many instances may be external and out of the control of the patient, and a therapeutic approach, which focuses on what the individual can do. That is, a CAM practitioner, like a biomedical practitioner, is unlikely to advise the patient to deal with the structural causes of cancer, such as polluted environments, but instead focus on what the individual patient can do, like search out and purchase what is usually more expensive organic food that might be less affected by the polluted environment.

CAM and the subaltern

In response to human suffering, people will draw on a range of therapeutic approaches. In most countries, a sanctioned cancer diagnosis can only be made by a medical doctor. Biomedicine is likely to be to the fore when it comes to responding to cancer, but alternative approaches are also likely to be sought out. In this section, I will consider the issue of medicinal cannabis being used by people with a diagnosis of cancer. The issue of medicinal cannabis brings some fascinating dimensions of the CAM/biomedicine tension to the fore. Medical cannabis has an ambiguous status. Cannabis can be a healing agent and also a drug of recreation, which is illegal in many countries and states. There have been clinical trials of synthesised forms of cannabis and these forms can be prescribed by medical doctors in many countries. Medicinal cannabis can also operate in subaltern forms, away from the purview of the state and of its functionaries, the medical profession.

For medicinal cannabis to gain state support, through such means as being evaluated as a safe medication and potentially subsidised by the state, then the formal channels of statist medicine must be appealed to, which means the 'alternative' treatment has to be reshaped into an acceptable form to statist medicine. Covert therapeutics, or what I refer to here as subaltern therapeutics, can also be administered, but with the threat of the state regulatory apparatus hanging over those who take such action.

In New Zealand, a debate over medicinal cannabis erupted in 2015 when a mother attempted to access medicinal cannabis for her hospitalised son (for a fuller discussion of this case, see Dew and Armstrong n.d.). This debate involved many players from different parts of the social, political and cultural spectrum of New Zealand, and new links were forged between a once forbidden drug and potentially beneficial health, economic and social effects.

The term medicinal cannabis can usefully be considered as a hybrid term. It brings together the status and credibility of the medical establishment and the deviant subculture of illicit drug consumption. If medicinal cannabis is to be tamed and reconfigured as a conventional therapeutic possibility, it must be distanced from subaltern therapeutics and embedded in systems of oversight and control that preserve the therapeutic status quo. The taming of medicinal cannabis is achieved through the extraction of specific ingredients from the plant that can be carefully controlled for dosage and potency, and that can then be put through the rigours of RCTs to determine efficacy (Grinspoon 2018). Cannabis contains over 500 compounds and there are over 100 cannabinoids (Elsohly et al. 2016). As this process of extraction and synthesis develops the therapeutic use of cannabis continues in subaltern forms, out of public view, in an unruly manner. In the subaltern, preference may be had for whole herb approaches to cannabis therapeutics, based on ideas of whole plant synergy and entourage effects that, amongst other purported benefits, can improve absorption and reduce side effects (Ben-Shabat et al. 1998).

The idea of subaltern therapeutic practices is noted in Chapter 6 in relation to a range of practices in South Asia. The term subaltern is derived from neo-Marxist analyses of hegemony. Antonio Gramsci used the term subaltern in relation to groups or collectives who are subject to the activity of ruling groups, even in situations of resistance. For Gramsci, the focus on class struggle and the contestation of hegemonic practices are not simply within the sphere of production, but can include other forms such as ecological, nationalist and religious ones (Morton 2007).

The term subaltern therapeutics has been taken up by South-Asian social science scholars to describe those everyday practices, sometimes labelled folk medicine, that evade and distance themselves from statist medicine (Hardiman and Mukharji 2012). Medicinal cannabis as a subaltern therapeutic practice has the additional alterity of being associated with the criminal world, and as such, in an environment of criminalised production and consumption of cannabis, must remain underground, evasive and distant. However, with sufficient emphasis on the medical aspect of medicinal cannabis it can become incorporated into statist biomedicine. Those players who are already organised and embedded within statist medicine can take medicinal cannabis as an object that is shaped by their own understandings, and it is put to work to bolster their own positions. Once incorporated into statist medicine, medicinal cannabis is divorced from the therapeutic practices in its subaltern form, shifting control from patients and subaltern practitioners to medical elites.

The case of medicinal cannabis complicates the picture, and even the concept, of therapeutic pluralism. Forms of cannabis that are refined, synthesised and standardised can be incorporated, or subsumed, into biomedicine, but only on biomedical terms. We can get then an expansion of therapeutic options within biomedicine, but perhaps at the cost of constraining actual therapeutic pluralism of the subaltern form if the production and supply of medicinal cannabis in the subaltern goes into decline.

As noted in Chapter 6, when I use the term statist medicine I am referring to the practices and organisations of biomedicine and the state regulatory apparatus in which it is entangled. The state apparatus includes the legal and regulatory systems that place prohibitions around who can diagnose and prescribe and what kinds of claims can be made about therapeutic practices. It also includes the processes of the approval of therapeutic products and the determinations of what products and services can be subsidised or funded by the state. The state apparatus varies across time and place, but important elements of it include the capacity of the medical profession to exclude its rivals, as discussed in Chapter 2, the requirements of the state to oversee health practices, and the role of commercial interests in state arrangements, particularly the role of drug companies (Dew 2003; Dew 2018; Freidson 1970; Larkin 1983; Willis 1983).

In its most subaltern phase, medicinal cannabis may have no visible centre or representative organisation. It operates through networks of people passing on information to each other, putting people in need in touch with those who can supply and so on. With the debates around the world and events related to the decriminalisation or legalisation of cannabis, visible organisations can appear to represent or advocate for those who access, or would like to access, cannabis products for therapeutic purposes, not necessarily in their synthesised form.

The material discussed later in this section comes from New Zealand, which at the time of writing had not followed many other states in the United States and other countries in the legalisation of recreational cannabis, that was initiated in 2012 when the states of Colorado and Washington passed laws to legalise cannabis (Shi et al. 2019).

Between legalisation and prohibition of the use of cannabis are situations where access to medicinal cannabis is allowed for certain conditions and licenses are provided for the production of cannabis for medical purposes. Such a situation has existed in Israel since the 1990s (Zarhin et al. 2018). In this circumstance, demarcations are required to determine whether a patient is a deserving recipient of a therapeutic intervention or is attempting to obtain cannabis for recreational purposes. In Israel, the Ministry of Health regulates the use of medicinal cannabis, and since 2007, it has been illegal for patients to grow cannabis. The production of cannabis for medical purposes is left to licensed commercial growers, and cannabis is only approved as a last resort for patients after other therapeutic options have failed, except for its use in treating the side effects of chemotherapy (Zarhin et al. 2018). Plans are also afoot in Israel to limit the use of medicinal cannabis to standardised product (Zarhin et al. 2018).

It is possible that the initial bottleneck created by statist medicine's regulatory processes, which limit access to unapproved subaltern practices, would eventually be undermined in the event of full legalisation of cannabis as these unapproved practices could be taken up by alternative health practitioners, as well as by folk who are not professionally trained. While this outcome may not be ideal from a state funding perspective, given the lower status of alternative medicine within the statist regime, it does point to an avenue for achieving the wider goals of subaltern patients and practitioners, whose practices will not always, or may never, meet the RCT gold standard claimed as the gateway to credibility by statist medicine (see Chapter 3). This situation might foster a greater level of therapeutic pluralism. On the other hand, the efforts towards making illegal non-standardised forms of medicinal cannabis in Israel points to a state response that may then leave access to subaltern forms as the only alternative for those who might not be able to afford state supplied products or who believe whole plant forms or other non-standardised forms offer greater therapeutic value.

The illegal status of cannabis was an issue in New Zealand that faced people who wanted to use it for medical purposes. In the popular imaginary, the distribution of cannabis may be associated with criminals, gangs and drug dealers. A new kind of supplier developed to distribute cannabis for medical use that provided some rhetorical distance from these popular negative associations – the suppliers were called green fairies. Green fairies are those who provide cannabis for therapeutic, not recreational, purposes. They are not labelled in the subaltern world as dealers, and so have attempted to create some distance from the negative connotations of dealers.

One green fairy was Rose Renton, whose son's time in hospital in 2015 gained a great deal of media coverage as Renton attempted to get doctors to prescribe cannabis for her son who had extreme seizures as a result of status epilepticus. Renton continued to fight for access to medicinal cannabis and act as a proponent of cannabis reform after the death of her son in hospital. In 2016, she delivered a 17,000-signature petition to parliament calling for the legalisation of medicinal cannabis, then in 2017 she was prosecuted for the possession and growing of cannabis in her role as a green fairy for her community.

Prominent citizens also lobbied for access to cannabis for medical purposes, such as Helen Kelly, then President of the Council of Trade Unions. She revealed to the media that she had been accessing cannabis illegally to self-medicate for pain while undergoing chemotherapy treatment for cancer. She tried and failed to gain access to medicinal cannabis through an application to the Associate Minister of Health and the Ministry of Health. Her advocacy efforts included support of the group Medical Cannabis Awareness New Zealand (MCANZ), which was established in 2016 to provide financial and other support for patients seeking access to the cannabis plant. Kelly died from cancer in late 2016.

During the start of this prominent media coverage in 2015, access to medicinal cannabis could be obtained through statist medicine, but at quite a price. The Ministry of Health had approved some drugs, like Sativex used for epilepsy, but the drug could only be accessed if ministerial approval was gained, which was a laborious bureaucratic hurdle to overcome. In addition, the drugs were not subsidised and so the costs were prohibitive for most people. So, even with the ninety-seven ministerial approvals obtained in 2015, there were only twenty-seven users of medicinal cannabis at that time, a disparity at least in part explained by the difficulty faced by potential users in funding the drug.

For some, staying within the legal or formal process of obtaining medicinal cannabis could be driven by fear of losing their jobs if they were caught engaging with the cannabis black market or concerns about having a consistent and standardised product. They would have to have the financial wherewithal to sustain purchasing the synthesised and state-approved products that were much more expensive than black market products.

Several reviews of the guidelines for approving cannabis were undertaken; however, all these reviews looked only at the possibility of freeing up access to cannabis as a pharmaceutical product and not access to those wanting whole herb cannabis or to use other cannabis products such as oils for therapeutic purposes. Some liberalising occurred, such as allowing medical specialists to make the call on prescribing to patients who are in the final stages of a terminal illness, as opposed to the Ministry of Health having to make the call. The government also changed legislation in order that cannabis products without psychoactive effects were reclassified, so that they would not be classed as a controlled drug under the Misuse of Drugs Act. However, concerns were raised within the medical profession that the system needed to change, so that it stopped sending patients to drug dealers (not labelled as green fairies in this context) by restricting access to medicinal cannabis. It was reported that up to sixty percent of cancer patients would be using cannabis illegally.

The unfolding of the debate over medicinal cannabis brings into sharp relief the existence of subaltern therapeutic forms. The operation and actions of the medical and legal complexes limit the public life of subaltern forms. The positioning of the medical profession and statist medicine in the face of subaltern therapeutic practices, the latter aligning with notions of patient empowerment and patient-centred care, was to reinforce the channels of standard assessment, eschewing any engagement with something like 'whole herb' therapeutics, and rather working through state agencies like the Ministry of Health to reassert biomedical hegemony.

The appearance of subaltern cancer therapeutic practices was a relatively brief one in New Zealand. Once access to synthesised forms was freed up, although not state subsidised, the subaltern practices gained less media attention, continuing as unseen forms of resistance. The unruly hybrid of medicinal cannabis has been, in practice, purified once again into the different and separate spaces of statist medicine and subaltern therapeutics. In the subaltern world, the production, distribution and consumption of therapeutic cannabis continues, with information shared in undocumented forms, dosages and procedures prescribed by unregulated 'therapists', and consumption based on trust and not official forms of credibility and status. In statist medicine, bureaucratic processes prevail but leave intact the control of the standardised form of therapeutic practice in medical hands. This is not to say, however, that standardised forms in medical hands eradicate the hybrid nature of medicinal cannabis. In clinical practice, where medicinal cannabis is an available option, there remain difficulties for clinicians to distinguish recreational use from medicinal use, and for some clinicians, the lack of scientific evidence for its efficacy remains an obstacle to prescription even in environments where it is legally available (Zolotov et al. 2018). In US research back in 2003 and 2004, over twenty-eight percent of medical doctors treating cancer patients supported the use of cannabis, but only 2.4 percent of patients were using it (Roberts et al. 2006). Clinicians in different specialities are more or less willing to prescribe it, for example, palliative care physicians being more open to prescribing a medication that is potentially addictive, drawing on their own observations and patient testimonials rather than relying on the science (Zolotov et al. 2018). In the subaltern realm, efforts to standardise potencies and experiment with different cannabis varieties occurs, drawing on the science rhetoric of statist medicine (Klein and Potter 2018).

The situation of the subaltern therapeutics of medicinal cannabis plays out in this way in New Zealand because of the status of cannabis as a criminalised object. If cannabis is legalised or decriminalised, then the subaltern practices of medicinal cannabis are likely to change. Although some people in the debate claimed that medicinal cannabis should be used as a whole herb, there was little in the way of the voices of herbalists, naturopaths or others practicing alternative health approaches. These practitioners sit somewhere between statist medicine and subaltern medicine, with some alternative therapists like chiropractors and osteopaths having regulatory recognition and state support through such things as state subsidies of student education, and others unregulated and without state support but operating openly (Dew 2003). If cannabis is legalised for recreational use, which is a real possibility, it is possible that practitioners of CAM may take on a more public role in advocating for the use of medicinal cannabis in ways that defy biomedical prescriptions. Or it is possible that statist medicine will maintain its hegemonic position by proscribing the claims that can be made about medicinal cannabis, so that any claims align with the outcomes of the formal regulatory processes of statist medicine – such as approval by the USA Food and Drug Administration and approval by MedSafe in New Zealand.

Another prominent set of actors in this therapeutic tussle are those who may profit from the legal production and distribution of cannabis products. Statist medicine can potentially be undermined by private interests pursuing profit, which in turn can benefit the state in terms of tax revenues and a potential reduction in the importation of pharmaceuticals with which medicinal cannabis would compete. The economic interests of the state may then provide a source of credibility and legitimacy for cannabis without going through the hoops of statist medicine's regulatory systems. An analogous situation occurred in China in relation to Tibetan medicine. In China, market reforms introduced in the post-Mao period impacted upon the provision of Tibetan medicine. Tibetan medical practices could be provided at low cost, with many medications produced from locally available materials. The evaluation of Tibetan medicine within the confines of statist medicine's regulatory frameworks was replaced by an assessment of Tibetan medicine based on its capacity to support economic development goals (Janes 2002). The same logic has the potential to play out in New Zealand and other countries if economic and patient interest groups could successfully combine forces.

Embedding medicinal cannabis into statist medicine would place economic as well as therapeutic constraints around its use. It would require isolated compounds of the cannabis plant being tested for safety and efficacy through the expensive process of RCTs, a process that requires capital investment (Yusuf et al. 2008). Subaltern economics is undertaken on a smaller scale, with producers and distributors not having such major capital outlay, and so enabling access to the plant and its products at a much lower price. However, in the subaltern space, the state does not provide any funding, whereas in statist medicine the possibilities of state subsidies have the potential to enable wider access.

The debates around medicinal cannabis may be unique as part of its subaltern positioning is a result of the illegal status of the plant as a drug of abuse. Information exchanges occur in informal ways, through such mechanisms as cannabis clubs (Klein and Potter 2018). But where claims about therapeutic outcomes are proscribed by statist medicine there are likely to be other forms of subaltern therapeutics. For example, proscribing what people can claim about a therapeutic practice may lead to the formation of information sharing practices that evade the gaze of the state, such as the use of closed or invitation only sites on social media. So, although the subaltern status of cannabis therapeutics is specific, its existence alerts us to the possibilities of other subaltern therapeutic practices.

Concluding comments

In the last chapter, we noted how patients negotiated their way through therapeutic options when responding to health issues. We see this here in much sharper form with cancer, where the stakes are higher, the options can be more drastic and the potential for conflict between health practitioners and patients is greater.

CAM use is high in cancer patients. But CAM has an ambiguous place in medicine. It is acceptable if it does not pose any epistemological or authoritative challenge to biomedicine, where it can be emphasised as complementary. Meditation, exercise and even prayer may be acceptable as they do not impinge upon treatment, especially if offered in hospice settings as opposed to hospital settings. CAM therapeutics are also acceptable if they can be transformed into a biomedical framing, as with synthesised forms of cannabis. The efforts of statist medicine to control cancer patients can be extreme, as in instances of forcing children to undertake biomedical cancer treatments against the will of parents. The state takes on the role of parent. CAM can however be allowed by biomedical practitioners in situations where biomedicine has nothing clear to offer.

The patient experience of CAM is, unsurprisingly, varied. CAM can be perceived to help ease anxieties, or it can be a desperate search for a cure or an extension of time. CAM users may assess its value in different ways from CAM and biomedical practitioners. Similarly, CAM practitioners inevitably hold a variety of views, as CAM itself is so varied. They may have complex understandings of cancer causation but may focus on the individual. This gives rise to concerns amongst social scientists that CAM fosters unrealistic hope and can blame the individual for getting cancer, or not being able to cure it. Medicinal cannabis provides hope of comfort for some. In the face of difficult or intolerable circumstances, many are willing to take the risk of using it even with its illegal status.

This complex relationship between biomedicine, CAM and patients with cancer results from the challenge to all of them that cancer poses. Biomedicine has gone down the track of using extremely toxic or radical treatments as the common line of intervention for cancer. This is daunting for patients. In many instances, this toxic approach is only aimed at extending life and not cure. The patient is faced with the possibility of a terminal diagnosis and the prospect of pain and extreme discomfort. The CAM practitioner might offer something different, ranging from assisting with the existential crisis that a cancer diagnosis can create to offering extreme alternatives in terms of dietary change and other aspects of regimen. But in doing so, they are potentially targeted for taking advantage of the vulnerable. Therapeutic possibilities are many, but in many instances, the choices are fraught. A therapeutic pluralism is extremely muted in cancer care from a biomedical perspective, but therapeutic hybridisation combining CAM and biomedicine is common for cancer patients.

References

Bell, K. (2010) Cancer survivorship, mor(t)ality and lifestyle discourses on cancer prevention, *Sociology of Health and Illness*, 32, 3, 349–364.

Ben-Shabat, S., Fride, E., Sheskin, T., Tamiri, T., Rhee, M.-H., Vogel, Z., Bisogno, T., De Petrocellis, L., Di Marzo, V. and Mechoulam, R. (1998) An entourage effect: Inactive endogenous fatty acid glycerol esters enhance 2-arachidonoyl-glycerol cannabinoid activity, *European Journal of Pharmacology*, 353, 1, 23–31.

Broom, A. (2000) *Boundary work: The construction of boundaries between 'alternative' and 'conventional' cancer treatments in New Zealand*, M.A. thesis, Christchurch: University of Canterbury.

——— (2006) Reflections on the centrality of power in medical sociology: An empirical test and theoretical elaboration, *Health Sociology Review*, 15, 5, 496–505.

Broom, A., Doron, A. and Tovey, P. (2009) The inequalities of medical pluralism: Hierarchies of health, the politics of tradition and the economies of care in Indian oncology, *Social Science & Medicine*, 69, 698–706.

Broom, A. and Tovey, P. (2007) Therapeutic pluralism? Evidence, power and legitimacy in UK cancer services, *Sociology of Health and Illness*, 29, 4, 551–569.

——— (2008) Exploring the temporal dimension in cancer patients' experiences of non-biomedical therapeutics, *Qualitative Health Research*, 18, 12, 1650–1661.

Chamberlain, K., Madden, H., Gabe, J., Dew, K. and Norris, P. (2011) Forms of resistance to medication within New Zealand households, *Medische Anthroplogie*, 23, 2, 299–308.

Cunningham, A., Phillips, C., Lockwood, G., Hedley, D. and Edmonds, C. (2000) Association of involvement in psychological self-regulation with longer survival in patients with metastatic cancer: An exploratory study, *Advances in Mind-Body Medicine*, 16, 4, 276–286.

Dew, K. (2003) *Borderland practices: Regulating alternative therapies in New Zealand*, Dunedin: University of Otago Press.

——— (2018) *Public health, personal health and pills: Drug entanglements and pharmaceuticalised governance*, London and New York: Routledge.

Dew, K. and Armstrong, L. (n.d.) Can the subaltern heal? Medical marijuana in Aotearoa New Zealand, *Journal of Sociology*, 10.1177/1440783320925144.

Dew, K., Signal, L., Davies, C., Tavite, H., Hooper, C., Safati, D., Stairmand, J. and Cunningham, C. (2015a) Dissonant roles: The experience of Māori in cancer care, *Social Science & Medicine*, 138, 144–151.

Dew, K., Signal, L., Stairmand, J., Simpson, A. and Sarfati, D. (2019) Cancer care decision-making and treatment consent: An observational study of patients' and clinicians' rights, *Journal of Sociology*, 55, 1, 161–178.

Dew, K., Stubbe, M., Signal, L., Stairmand, J., Dennett, E., Koea, J., Simpson, A., Sarfati, D., Cunningham, C., Batten, L., Ellison-Loschmann, L., Barton, J. and Holdaway, M. (2015b) Cancer care decision making in multidisciplinary meetings, *Qualitative Health Research*, 25, 3, 397–407.

Elsohly, M.A., Mehmedic, Z., Foster, S., Gon, C., Chandra, S. and Church, J.C. (2016) Changes in cannabis potency over the last 2 decades (1995–2014): Analysis of current data in the United States, *Biological Psychiatry*, 79, 7, 613–619.

Freidson, E. (1970) *Profession of medicine: A study of the sociology of applied knowledge*, New York: Dodd, Mead.

Grinspoon, P. (2018) Cannabidiol (CBD): What we know and what we don't, *Harvard Health Blog*, www.health.harvard.edu/blog/cannabidiol-cbd-what-we-know-and-what-we-dont-2018082414476.

Hansen, F., Berntsen, G.R. and Salamonsen, A. (2020) Medical pluralism in the aftermath of cancer health seeking actions and cancer patients' shaping of trajectories to healing, *Anthropology & Medicine*, 27, 3, 330–346.

Hardiman, D. and Mukharji, P.B. (2012) *Medical marginality in South Asia: Situating subaltern therapeutics*, London: Routledge.

Hök, J., Forss, A., Falkenberg, T. and Tishelman, C. (2009) What is an exceptional cancer trajectory?: Multiple stakeholder perspectives on cancer trajectories in relation to complementary and alternative medicine use, *Integrative Cancer Therapies*, 8, 2, 153–163.

Janes, C. (2002) Buddhism, science, and market: The globalisation of Tibetan medicine, *Anthropology & Medicine*, 9, 3, 267–289.

Klein, A. and Potter, G. (2018) The three betrayals of the medical cannabis growing activist: From multiple victimhood to reconstruction, redemption and activism, *The International Journal on Drug Policy*, 53, 65.

Larkin, G. (1983) *Occupational monopoly and modern medicine*, London: Tavistock Press.

Molassiotis, A., Fernadez-Ortega, P., Pud, D., Ozden, G., Scott, J.A., Panteli, V., Margulies, A., Browall, M., Magri, M., Selvekerova, S., Madsen, E., Milovics, L., Bruyns, I., Gudmundsdottir, G., Hummerston, S., Ahmad, A.M.A., Platin, N., Kearney, N. and Patiraki, E. (2005) Use of complementary and alternative medicine in cancer patients: A European survey, *Annals of Oncology*, 16, 4, 655–663.

Morton, A.D. (2007) *Unravelling Gramsci: Hegemony and passive revolution in the global political economy*, London: Pluto Press.

Olson, R. (2015) *Towards a sociology of cancer caregiving: Time to feel*, Farnham: Ashgate.

Roberts, C.S., Baker, F., Hann, D., Runfola, J., Witt, C., McDonald, J., Livingston, M.L., Ruiterman, J., Ampela, R., Kaw, O.C. and Blanchard, C. (2006) Patient-physician communication regarding use of complementary therapies during cancer treatment, *Journal of Psychosocial Oncology*, 23, 4, 35–60.

Sered, S. and Agigian, A. (2008) Holistic sickening: Breast cancer and the discursive worlds of complementary and alternative practitioners, *Sociology of Health & Illness*, 30, 4, 616–631.

Shi, Y., Liang, D., Bao, Y., An, R., Wallace, M.S. and Grant, I. (2019) Recreational marijuana legalization and prescription opioids received by Medicaid enrollees, *Drug and Alcohol Dependence*, 194, 13–19.

Tovey, P. and Broom, A. (2008) The problematic nature of conflating use and advocacy in CAM integration: Complexity and differentiation in UK cancer patients' views, *Health Sociology Review*, 17, 4, 384–395.

Willis, E. (1983) *Medical dominance: The division of labour in Australian healthcare*, Sydney: George Allen & Unwin.

Yusuf, S., Bosch, J., Devereaux, P., Collins, R., Baigent, C., Granger, C., Califf, R. and Temple, R. (2008) Sensible guidelines for the conduct of large randomized trials, *Clinical Trials*, 5, 1, 38–39.

Zarhin, D., Negev, M., Vulfsons, S. and Sznitman, S.R. (2018) Rhetorical and regulatory boundary-work: The case of medical cannabis policy-making in Israel, *Social Science & Medicine*, 217, 1–9.

Zolotov, Y., Vulfsons, S., Zarhin, D. and Sznitman, S. (2018) Medical cannabis: An oxymoron? Physicians' perceptions of medical cannabis, *International Journal of Drug Policy*, 57, 4–10.

9

INCOHERENT FORCES

The disciplining and the unruliness of complementary and alternative therapies

In the introduction, I suggested that therapeutic pluralism is more or less available at the level of the household, the level of the clinic and the practitioner, the level of the professional organisation and the level of the state and its regulations, and indeed, at the level of something broader and more ephemeral, that of the culture of a society. Therapeutic pluralism may be embraced or descried. The latter position can be seen in this quote from a 1923 Government of Madras report on indigenous systems of medicine.

> The rate at which specialists of this type are increasing is truly appalling. One would cure all ills by osteopathy, another by chromopathy, another by homeopathy, a fourth by allopathy, others by electricity, baths, food reform, vaccine-therapy, charms, incantation, miracle workings, magnetic healing . . . the list goes on. . . . It is only natural that under such circumstances, a sort of distrust of all specialists is created in the popular mind.
>
> *(cited in Bivins 2007: 155)*

The choice of therapeutic approaches is even more extensive now than it was in 1923. How CAM therapies and biomedicine (or allopathy in the above quote) relate and what therapies should be sanctioned have been sources of contention for a long time. Through examining different levels of healthcare-related activity, conflicting forces can be seen. What forces come to the fore are dependent on the particulars of the local context that is shaped by social, political, technological, scientific, environmental and ideological elements, amongst others.

The idea of orthodoxy and its alternatives is not pregiven. It is constructed and becomes manifest through interactions between people whether in consultations rooms, at commissions of inquiry, in front of policy makers or in homes. In the opening chapters of this book, the constraining and limiting influences on therapeutic possibilities were emphasised. In the West, therapeutic identities were solidified from the mid-nineteenth century when the profession of medicine attained control over who could be called a medical doctor. In doing so, the boundaries between alternative medicine and orthodox medicine could be more clearly policed. The state-regulated medical organisations could determine who was to be given the status and privileges of a medical doctor and who was not. The medical profession was now firmly entwined with the state, and the development and evolution of statist medicine was now in train.

Statist medicine transformed through technological and methodological developments and changes to the way disease, bodies and healing was understood. The individual patient as a singular unit of attention was decentred. On the one hand, laboratory medicine and new medical instruments fragmented the patient, reducing the patient to a diagnostic category. What was found from laboratory results, what could be heard through stethoscopes, what could be seen on cardiograms and so on was now a central focus of medical work. On the other hand, the individual patient was subsumed into the population of all people with like signs and symptoms, and the treatment to prescribe could be identified through the RCT. Technological and methodological developments in biomedicine became increasingly standardised, as the state sought to rein in healthcare costs and foster greater levels of trust in the medical profession. Trust in numbers was the means to achieve this, with auditing, guidelines and new disciplinary procedures constraining the autonomy of the individual medical practitioner, in turn limiting the range of therapeutic possibilities that could be on offer in the doctor patient encounter.

Biomedicine strives to shape CAM practices in its own image (Brosnan et al. 2018). It can attempt to achieve this in many ways. CAM interventions can be acceptable to biomedicine if they can jump the hurdle of the RCT, as long as the effects of CAM can be explained in biomedical terms. There are examples of CAM therapies attaining this goal, such as acupuncture in certain conditions, including the treatment of mental illness (Roberts et al. 2020). Biomedicine can attempt to identify a specific therapeutic compound from an alternative botanical treatment, and once identified synthesise the compound for mass production of medications, as with extracts from medical cannabis. Trials and drug development of this nature are based on assumptions of needing standardised treatments for standardised populations. In some settings, biomedicine can assimilate CAM practices alongside its own, such as meditation practices in hospices. Assimilation, or integration, can operate as a mechanism of biomedical dominance as practices are incorporated in ways that do not challenge biomedical practices, biomedical understandings and biomedical authority.

Therapeutic practices are shaped in spheres where CAM practices engage with state or state-sanctioned institutions. Inside universities where CAM courses may be available, they are likely to be taught on the basis of biomedical science. Where research is undertaken it is on the terms of biomedical research. And even in these situations, those who dare to take CAM seriously may come under harsh attack from the media for entertaining pseudoscience, a position uncritically taken up by journalists from apologist medical groups defending the boundaries of orthodox therapeutic practice.

From this reading, there is a social trend of increasingly limited therapeutic possibilities inside the medical profession. This has impacted on those outside the medical profession offering therapeutic services. The case of chiropractic illustrates this. Chiropractic has endeavoured to gain access to some of the resources available to the medical profession. In making its case for access, it has had to claim that it is a distinct profession that can do something that the medical profession cannot do or cannot do so well. In doing so, it has to maintain a delicate balance. With the medical professions' understanding of therapeutics having hegemonic status, chiropractic could not challenge medicine by offering a different approach to therapeutics. To do so would now be seen as irrational, radical and unconscionable. And so, chiropractic gave up its claim to be a universal therapeutic approach. Despite chiropractic receiving overwhelming support from US courts and in other fora such as in state inquiries, and the medical profession being vilified for its efforts to suppress it, chiropractic was to be limited in its claims, so that it did not challenge the cultural authority of biomedicine. This process of limitation is further enhanced with increasing institutional acceptance. In the United Kingdom and Australia, where chiropractic is taught in some universities, there is evidence of chiropractic academics distancing themselves from the therapies vitalist philosophies, pushing to make chiropractic more evidence-based using biomedical methodological forms, and reframing the therapy from offering an alternative health system to being allied to health, and in the long run unlikely to be distinguishable from physiotherapy (Brosnan 2017).

Counter to this journey of therapeutic limitations, there are other tendencies that may open up or maintain therapeutic possibilities. One is the limitations on the control over individual medical practitioners, despite the trends of the medical profession to increasingly govern its membership through re-licensing, auditing and disciplining mechanisms. CAM still has a hold inside of the medical profession. Efforts at providing integrative health services speak to this desire. Yet on closer examination, integrative health services may be less about embracing therapeutic possibilities and more about constraining the impact of CAM by dominating it. It is better to have popular CAM approaches inside biomedicine where they can be overseen and restrained, rather than outside pulling patients away. This is one strand of the argument made by medical acupuncturists to promote themselves as a legitimate grouping within biomedicine. Jon Adams' discussion of boundary work is relevant, with medical practitioners who use CAM establishing rhetorical boundaries between themselves and lay practitioners, but also doing similar work in relation to their own practices and the rhetorical claims to evidence-based medicine of their medical colleagues (Adams 2004). He also notes in his discussion of GPs who use CAM in the United Kingdom that they may take contradictory positions depending on what was being talked about and who the audience was (Adams 2004). The case of medical acupuncturists clearly shows this happening, and also it is likely that once biomedical practitioners engage with CAM practices, like acupuncture, some may be lured into a deeper involvement in theoretical and practice concerns that challenge biomedicine. They may, for example, consider the utility of concepts used in Chinese medicine, or seriously ask questions about the role of intuition or other 'irrational' components of therapeutic practice.

Although biomedicine now underpins statist medicine throughout the globe, there are situations where statist medicine itself can foster greater therapeutic possibilities. This is most clearly evident in countries where fully developed therapeutic systems were in operation prior to incursions of Western medicine, such as in China and India. The ebb and flow of the legitimation of Chinese medicine in China and the many therapeutic traditions in India, particularly ayurveda, unani tibb, siddha and sowa rigpa, are not based on definitive scientific evidence, but the changing ideologies and needs of the state. The status of traditional medicine waxed and waned in response to imperialism and nationalism. Traditional medicines could claim science, but a different science from that which underpins biomedicine. The past could be revered rather than abjured. But for all the continuity with the past traditional medicines evolve, in their teaching, practices and research, in relation to biomedicine, to each other and to broader political, economic and social developments. Therapeutic pluralism is close to being realised when the state supports other therapeutic practices besides biomedicine, but the evolution of these other therapeutic practices is moulded by standardising processes and the methodological underpinnings of biomedicine when these practices come into the state orbit.

Outside of the state orbit is an array of subaltern, folk and everyday practices, both in non-Western societies and in the West. In China, the subaltern may operate in the household, but also in the master-disciple relationship where therapeutic practices are passed on, beyond standardising mechanisms and the glare of the state apparatus. In India, tribal healers, bonesetters and localised therapeutic regimens like chandshir operate in ways unregulated by the state, but firmly embedded in communities and villages.

Folk and subaltern practices thrive in the West as well. The folk medicine in the United States can look very similar at times to the folk medicine practiced in South Asia discussed in Chapter 6. For example, herbalists in the Appalachians passed their knowledge down through the generations. In some parts of America, people consulted with the 'Old Lady', someone who advises on the treatment of ordinary illnesses but does not have consulting rooms or office hours (Baer 2001). Folk medicine practices could combine divine healing and home remedies. African American folk medicine could be highly syncretic combining aspects of voodoo, Christian healing practices, herbs, charms and conjuring. Folk healers could also combine their healing practices with biomedicine, such as the Mexican American curanderos who could provide injections of vitamins or penicillin, with antibiotics purchased across the border from Mexican drug stores (Baer 2001).

The syncretic and subaltern nature of some practices can be captured in the following description of the working space of a Puerto Rican espiritismo practitioner, a madrina (godmother), that Hans Baer summarises from the work of ethnographers: 'a one-room storefront, which included the sanctuary, a small kitchen, a secluded healing area, and small botanica that sold healing and protective articles such as herbs, cleansing baths, candles, incense, and statues of the Catholic saints and Yoruba gods' (Baer 2001: 164).

There are many varieties of Native American healing systems. A well-known practice is the sweat lodge of the Plains Indians, where a small number of males gather, and a medicine man sprinkles water over heated stones to create a rush of hot air and the participants sing and pray. The lodges can be used to overcome physical ills and tackling such problems as addiction and alcoholism (Baer 2001). The Navajo Indians incorporate mythic sand paintings into their healing practices that symbolise the restoration of harmony (Baer 2001). The use of peyote, an import from Mexico, is used by the southern Plains tribes in curing ceremonies as well as a variety of other communal practices. The consumption of peyote is accompanied by prayers, singing and drumming, and has institutionalised and legally recognised support through the Native American Church (Baer 2001).

Navajo have different approaches to healing depending on what is regarded as the likely cause. Stephen Kunitz and Jerrold Levy (1997) suggest a division between disease, which is caused by such things as witchcraft or a breach of tabu and requires shamans or ceremonialists to remove the cause, and symptoms which could be treated by herbal remedies, setting bones, cauterisation and so on and could be undertaken by a knowledgeable person. Navajo make use of Western medicine, aligning it with the treatment of symptoms rather that disease, and may use ceremonials to effect a cure (Kunitz and Levy 1997). The links between religion and healing are strong, with 'singers', people whose knowledge of ritual is gained through apprenticeship, tasked with curing illness, and diviners who diagnose on the basis of an unsought gift of hand trembling (Kunitz and Levy 1997). The demanding apprenticeship of the ceremonialists has led to a drop in their availability, and since the 1950s, younger Navajo men have taken up the less demanding training in peyote ceremonialism instead, the latter more possible to attain for wage labourers (Kunitz and Levy 1997).

From this brief summary, it is evident that Western indigenous and folk practices are as diverse as those on the Indian subcontinent. Not only diverse, but syncretic and often combining religious and healing practices, or treating those practices as one and the same thing. These subaltern practices are evolving and changing in relation to each other and in response to broader social change. Throughout the globe, therapeutic practices take on a different hue inside households. In the West, the therapeutic activities in the household exhibit the medley of hybrid practices that are undisciplined by the mechanisms of statist medicine and the compulsions of CAM therapeutic practitioners. Householder mix and match CAM therapies, and combine CAM therapies with biomedicine, making therapeutic decisions based on their own understandings, observation and values. An attitude of epistemic eclecticism has been suggested to describe the ways in which people undertake therapeutic activities (Hornberger 2019). This suggests that people shift from one way of knowing to another as they draw on CAM or biomedical therapeutics. But perhaps epistemic agnosticism fits this better, or that people relegate epistemology to irrelevance in taking a pragmatic view about what works. Developments in statist medicine, CAM and subaltern practices provide the therapeutic canvas that people can draw on, but the image they create may not be envisioned by anyone.

The mixing, matching and blending of therapeutic practices confronts the stark possibilities of life-limiting illness in cancer care. A cancer diagnosis will very likely foster efforts to seek out care beyond biomedicine, sometimes in efforts to deal with the harsh interventions of biomedicine, sometimes to seek cure when biomedicine offers none and sometimes to deal with the existential issues faced by possible death, issues that biomedicine does not engage with. In cancer care, we see the range of possibilities for how CAM and biomedicine can interrelate, from a stance of complete opposition to efforts at some form of accommodation. The grave possibilities faced when a cancer diagnosis is made can even cultivate efforts to seek out illegal subaltern approaches, such as the use of medical cannabis. The status and perception of cannabis as a drug of recreation requires those who desire to acquire it to run the risk of legal challenge, a risk that many take when statist medicine obstructs access to desired therapeutic possibilities.

Much of the debate about CAM relates to understandings of science and whether CAM therapies have been or can be successfully validated or not. Harry Collins and Trevor Pinch (Collins 1998) propose that all science is subject to the experimenter's regress. The experimenter's regress pivots around the question of what is the correct outcome of an experiment? If the answer is already known (like the boiling point of water), then one can determine whether there was something wrong with the experiment (contaminated water, incorrectly reading thermometer and so on) or not. If we do not know the outcome of the experiment, then there is no way of knowing if our experiment is a good one or a bad one. In any controversial issue, the outcome is not determined by experiments, but by a consensus. Any experiment that supports the consensus is hailed as a good experiment, competently carried out. Any experiment that goes against the consensus is deemed as faulty or carried out by incompetent experimenters or frauds. Any amount of data collected by medical acupuncturists or chiropractors could be dismissed if it did not conform to the views of the consensus. This consensus may have very little to do with science (Collins 1998). The acceptance of chiropractic and acupuncture was not based on the definitive scientific experiment which proved beyond all doubt that they worked. In both instances, a precarious balancing act had to be performed. For the medical acupuncturists and chiropractors, connections between their therapy and irrationalism had to be broken.

These examples highlight the ways in which different strategies can be invoked according to circumstances. It is not simply a matter of identifying some within acupuncture as being scientific and some as being unscientific. Science is called upon in different situations, and in other situations, science is seen as too limiting and constraining. Organisations and individuals do not necessarily adopt static positions, but their arguments are fluid and can change with the particular situation being confronted.

CAM only exists as a concept in relation to statist medicine. The relationship that CAM takes to statist medicine is incredibly varied. Therapeutic possibilities can be expanded or contracted in many different ways. Biomedicine can open itself up to CAM practices, as in integrative medicine that may expand what might be available to people in biomedical settings. Integrative medicine may contract therapeutic possibilities as CAM practices are redefined and re-described in biomedical terms. Biomedicine can vitriolically oppose CAM practices, as we see historically with homeopathy, chiropractic and in some cases where people with a cancer diagnosis choose CAM options. Suppression efforts do not necessarily work in ways anticipated as people seek out alternatives to dominant medical systems to find what works for them. Suppression can lead to unintended consequences such as patients not telling their biomedical practitioners what they are taking or doing for fear of disapproval, or patients avoiding biomedicine altogether. Medical practitioners themselves can be subjected to suppression efforts. In Portugal, a medical doctor risks being banned from practising medicine by the Medical Council if he or she claims to be a homeopath, or to practice homeopathy. So, those medical practitioners who have learnt homeopathy keep it a secret from the Medical Council (Almeida 2012). The suppression or integration of CAM are not the only options for relationships between CAM and biomedicine. Alternative approaches can co-exist with biomedicine, even at state level. Statist medicine can, in some cases, include approaches that are not biomedical, such as ayurveda and siddha medicine. In such circumstances, non-biomedical approaches may start to take the shape of biomedicine, most dramatically seen in the case of osteopathy in the United States.

CAM practices are dynamic, evolving and cannot be tied down as some sort of singular and homogenous approach. As Volker Scheid demonstrates for Chinese medicine and Jean Langford for ayurveda medicine, these systems and practices cannot be reduced to some singular total system, as therapeutic practices take on diverse faces, discourses and practices as manifestations of multiple influences, including individual practitioner understandings and positionings, professional pronouncements and the demands of the state. Scheid (2002) convincingly argues that plurality is just the way things are, with therapeutic practices in a constant process of change and transformation. There is no stable state of practice. Chinese medicine is not a system but a process. Scheid's conclusion from his detailed study of Chinese medicine and its history is applicable to all therapeutic practices, including biomedicine. Within the same named CAM therapy, there are an abundance of approaches. Medical acupuncture is not one entity, let alone TCM. There are opposing schools of thought and practice within chiropractic. There are many naturopathies. The multiplicity of therapeutic approaches is omnipresent. There are then a plurality of therapeutic options always available, but over time some of these are more visible than others, and some are given more legitimacy than others.

Therapeutic pluralism refers to both what is out there that can be selected from and what people do in practice. In practice, therapeutic pluralism is endemic, but the intensity varies based, in part, on the 'out there' availability and accessibility of therapeutic options. It is endemic in people's everyday healing and health-seeking practices, and arguably in the practice of those providing health services.

How patients, practitioners, organisations and states position alternative healing practices are incredibly variable. The variation is partly an outcome of opposing struggles to enhance or suppress alternative medicine. The relationship within CAM therapies, between different CAM therapies, and between CAM therapies and biomedicine can be abrasive. But the dynamic and evolving nature of therapeutic practices and their interactions with each other continue to create opportunities and options for those seeking solutions to illness, disease and disability. When people seek out therapeutic practices, they draw on a very wide range of sources of information, with biomedical and CAM practitioners being sources of authority amongst many others. And people do not passively accept the authority of healthcare practitioners, but actively engage in experimentation, observation and assessment of practices. From this perspective, there is then no simple notion of 'alternative' as inside households there is no orthodoxy. Therapeutic possibilities abound in undisciplined forms.

References

Adams, J. (2004) *Demarcating the medical/non-medical border: Occupational boundary-work within GPs' accounts of their integrative practice*, Abingdon, UK: Routledge.

Almeida, J. (2012) The differential incorporation of CAM into the medical establishment: The case of acupuncture and homeopathy in Portugal, *Health Sociology Review*, 765–792.

Baer, H. (2001) *Biomedicine and alternative healing systems in America: Issues of class, race, ethnicity and gender*, Madison: The University of Wisconsin Press.

Bivins, R. (2007) *Alternative medicine: A history*, Oxford: Oxford University Press.

Brosnan, C. (2017) Alternative futures: Fields, boundaries, and divergent professionalisation strategies within the Chiropractic profession, *Social Science & Medicine*, 190, 83–91.

Brosnan, C., Vuolanto, P. and Brodin Danell, J. (2018) Introduction: Reconceptualising complementary and alternative medicine as knowledge production and social transformation, in C. Brosnan, P. Vuolanto and J. Brodin Danell (eds.), *Complementary and alternative medicine knowledge production and social transformation*, Cham: Springer International Publishing, pp. 1–29.

Collins, H.M., Pinch, T. (1998) *The golem: What you should know about science*, Cambridge, England: Cambridge University Press.

Hornberger, J. (2019) Who is the fake one now? Questions of quackery, worldliness and legitimacy, *Critical Public Health*, 29, 4, 484–493.